TABLE OF CONTENTS

INTRODUCTION

This book was written to share my experience as a mother of three kids about breastfeeding and their initiation on a very important aspect of their lives as eating could be.

As a mother, I consider it essential to accompany them through this special journey to a healthy, both socially and nutritionally way to relate with food and its rituals.

A healthy diet does involve not only healthy ingredients and balanced nutrients in each meal, but also a healthy social interchange which will bring joy and a sense of belonging to any human being. We, parents, hold a very important responsibility throughout this process of making our kids enjoy food and learn to communicate during eating times.

Mealtime is a very important moment to develop life lasting habits, as cleaning their hands before and after eating, brushing their teeth after every meal, and acquiring good manners, to name a few examples.

I specially develop breastfeeding section because I consider it is the best gift you can give to your child, helping him develop not only a good immune system and a healthy growth but also the foundation of love and caregiving that would build their inner security in life later. Bottle feeding can also help develop this aspect, but believe me, it is not the same. So if you have the chance, breastfeed your baby as long as you can. Even a few months could make a big difference in your baby`s way to relate to his environment.

The other stages, important as they are, will introduce baby food recipes, classified by age and abilities, and some tips and advice I 'd been learning with my sons.

Cooking is a gift of love you can offer your kids every single day, so don't miss the possibility to give them a meal prepared with mum's loving and caring hands. I can assure taste is not the same when love is involved in the preparation of a kid's food. My kids have always pointed that at me.

Enjoy cooking for your kids. Even if you are a working mother as I Was, there is always a way to deal with problems and challenges, wearing a big smile, continuously learning in the process. Our kids deserve trying, and they can be very supportive. Ask for help if you need to, learn to lean on people who love you. And above all, enjoy being a mother!

I hope you find this book useful and practical. Have fun and be patient at yourself!

CHAPTER 1. BABY FOOD 101

Thinking about the growth of a small child involves their feeding directly, and it is not an easy task for us, parents, to make it a healthy way. That is why this book, divided into several chapters, shows how to translate the information we have about children's health and nutrition into substantial, attractive and physiologically adequate meals for age, cognitive and metabolic maturation at different ages, including recipes based on the main ingredients of each period, which, in turn, serve as triggers to make other nutritional variants.

The incorporation of new food must be varied and nutritious, as a way of helping children to spend their childhood trying different flavors and not only the three or four traditional dishes (French fries, hamburgers, hot dogs, etc.), that only lead them to behaviors such as capriciously rejecting other foods without even having tasted them. The phrase we have endlessly heard "I do not like it" has its origins on the lost opportunity to try new flavors at the right time.

Between the first five years of life, beginning to establish food preferences is very important to give our kids the chance to choose between different, healthy foods that allow them to eat well from a very young age. The variety of recipes proposed here for these years of life also contribute to the prevention of diseases such as obesity, high blood pressure, hypercholesterolemia, and diabetes, among others.

However, believe me when I tell you that it is not just about eating. As parents, we need to teach our children the habits and healthy eating and social behaviors that will mark them for life.

I desire to contribute to the development of a healthy childhood, with life habits that encourage family reunion around a table, and that favor the growth of the little ones, making the time to eat pleasant, full of joy and communication.

Introduce solids at about six months of age

Breast milk is an important food for babies until at least 12 months of age, or longer if the mum and baby desire. Infant formula is important until 12 months. By about six months of age, a baby's iron stores are low and extra foods will be needed to maintain healthy growth and prevent nutritional problems such as iron deficiency. Start by introducing solids around six months of age – when your baby starts showing interest in food.

BREASTFEEDING

Breastfeeding should be a gratifying aspect of baby care since you will be providing the best nutrition that nature is capable of the offering; Do not be discouraged if you find some problems in the first days. Both of you must learn together this new technique. Be patient if at first, your baby does not seem to know how to suck or doesn't do it for a long time. The child does not need to eat much immediately after birth, and your nipples take a while to become firm and get used to sucking.

Eating time for both mom and baby, should be a relaxing, reassuring and deeply happy experience.

From the first minutes of life, if your baby is vital and vigorous, you can put him to the breast. Early sucking of the nipples promotes detachment of the placenta and faster recovery of the usual uterine size. The blood vessels contract more quickly, decreasing bleeding. A hormone, oxytocin, is secreted each time the baby begins to suck. She is responsible for the changes described.

For the baby, the mother's milk is a source of nutrients, many of which are not found in any artificial milk.

It is better absorbed and digested and has the right temperature. Lactose, which is the milk sugar, contributes to the development of the intestinal flora and decreases gas and constipation. From the immunological point of view, breast milk provides many antibodies that protect the baby from infections (mainly intestinal and respiratory): breastfed infants suffer less frequently from viral and allergic diseases. Another advantage to be considered is that the newborn will receive from the breast a sterile food, at an adequate temperature, ready to be consumed. The baby will never be overfed or obese and will be protected against hypercholesterolemia.

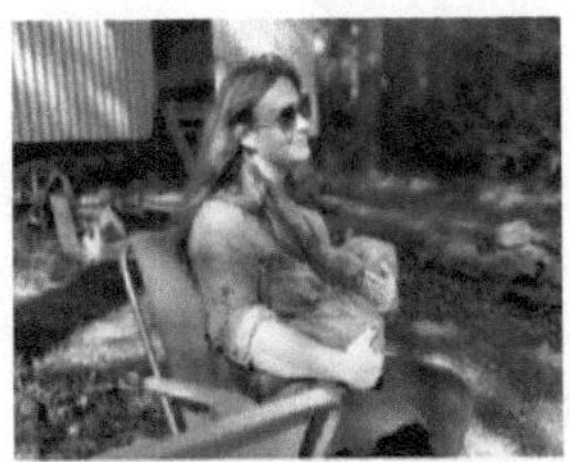

Sometimes, the simple fact of being near the baby, thinking about it or hearing it cry are enough causes for milk to spill from the nipples. This situation should not disturb mothers since it is normal. On the other hand, the states of concern or the fear of being inadequately feeding the baby determine the release of substances that can inhibit breastfeeding.

Colostrum

The first milk secretion is called colostrum. Characterized as a transparent yellowish liquid, of apparent lesser consistency than mature milk, this food with which the mother has endowed nature allows her to adequately nourish her baby in the first days when the intestine is not yet sufficiently mature enough to receive another type of milk. It contains a smaller proportion of carbohydrates and fats, and proteins and minerals are the predominant elements. Its high defensive power makes it the best contribution of antibodies to protect the baby against all types of infection. During the first days, frequent breastfeeding contributes to the appearance of mature milk and at the same time helps both the baby and the mother to adapt to this complex, but a not difficult, process called breastfeeding.

Reflection of descent of the milk

The descent of the milk is established between the fourth and the eighth day, preceded by a type of milk called intermediate that occurs after colostrum.

The stimulation produced by the suction of the baby in the nipple and areola sends a message to the brain, to secrete two hormones: oxytocin, which in addition to contributing to the contraction of the uterus contracts the breast alveoli allowing the milk to escape, and prolactin, which is responsible for the maintenance of breastfeeding. When the baby suckles the breast, squeezes the areola, the darkest area around the nipple; From this stimulus the brain sends a message to the mammary gland to produce milk. The milk penetrates the milk ducts and accumulates in the deposits behind the nipple, from where the baby can take it out in each feeding.

Composition of milk

• Breast milk shows unattainable differences concerning vegetable -soybean-, animal or formula milk, both in nutritional intake and in its immunological properties, protecting the baby from infections and allergic diseases.

• The volume and daily milk production are variable among women. It is considered that all breastfeeding mothers produce a volume of milk less than the secretory capacity of the mammary gland.

• The amount of milk that each mother generates daily is regulated by the demand of the baby and the suction-extraction that she makes in each feeding.

• The average volume of milk production is 600 to 900 ml per day. This excellent milk production capacity will remain until the food is introduced when it begins to decline.

• When the incorporation of food takes place around four months, this decline is very significant, whereas if it is done after six months, it will be possible to maintain a production greater than 500 ml per day for as long as you want to breastfeed the baby.

The nutrients

Proteins: have higher nutritional value, and better digestibility; Because they are of human origin, allergies that can be produced by the proteins found in cow's milk or formula are avoided.

Water: the baby's body is almost 80% made up of water. This percentage decreases as the child grows. The breast milk provides in each feeding the amount of water necessary to maintain this balance. The need is covered in every healthy baby that ingests around 200 cubic centimeters per kilo of weight and per day. This contribution should be supplemented with water when it is too hot; the baby transpires a lot or has a fever.

Fats: the content is variable between different people, and in each feeding. Its concentration can be higher in general and in the last part of milk. It also changes during the day (higher in the morning than in the evening).

Lactose: it is an indispensable source of energy. When transformed into lactic acid favors the absorption of minerals contained in breast milk (enough to meet the needs of the baby).

Vitamins: the mother needs a balanced diet to transfer to the baby the highest number of vitamins and micronutrients since some of them reduce the secretion by the mother's milk when they are insufficient in the feeding of the mother. The most significant are riboflavin, vitamin A, iodine, selenium, vitamin B6 and 612, while others such as vitamin D, calcium, iron, zinc, and copper are little modified in milk with maternal ingestion or supplement.

Modulators of growth: are biologically active substances that contribute to the production of hormones, such as growth.

Importance of breastfeeding

Today, unlike in the past, breastfeeding starts earlier. The baby is born knowing how to be fed. For this purpose, it has the suction and the search reflex. These reflexes will allow your baby to eat when hungry, but they are NOT indicators that the baby is hungry at all. If you pamper your baby on his cheeks or around his mouth, it will orient his face to the side of the stimulus. In the same way, this reflex will start if you put your finger or pacifier in your baby's mouth.

Until a schedule is established, the baby will be fed on demand, meaning that there are no rigid schedules to feed it. In this process of mutual learning, it will be advisable that you take an interval of two to four hours at most as a guide to breastfeeding your baby. At night you can let him sleep all he wants since at this time there are biological regulatory mechanisms that avoid that the baby can suffer some problems for not receiving milk.

It is a mistake to think that the baby can learn to eat with rigid schedules. For this reason, if you let him cry for too long, between breastfeeds, he will end up so tired that he will not have the strength to eat well. It is essential to satisfy the baby whenever he demands it, helping you organize the diet and avoid the side effects on dairy production. Remember: tranquility and time will be your best allies.

Breastfeeding creates a unique and indissoluble link between mother and son.

The suction time of each breast should be similar; in this way, the stimulus they receive to produce milk will be the same in both mammary glands. But also, if the mother wants it, she could breastfeed the baby with only one breast and reserve the other for the next breastfeed. Consider this as a good option for the first days, when the baby eats very often.

When the baby can establish pauses of three or four hours, it is convenient to divide the feeding time between the two breasts. The baby will be able to suckle between five and twenty minutes in each of the breasts. It is essential to establish a global feeding time to get a better organization of this process. For example: if it takes ten minutes from one breast and then six from the other, then the overall feeding time is sixteen minutes. This time is divided into two, and in the next feeding, start with the breast the baby finished eating for eight minutes. Then move the baby to the other breast to complete its feeding another eight minutes or whatever time the baby wants to. The global time is established again to restart the cycle in the next breastfeed.

In this way, you will make an even extraction of the two breasts, and therefore there will be an adequate replacement in both, as Inexperienced nipples better tolerate short, frequent breastfeeds. The more practice you get, the easier it will be when your baby starts to suck hard. You can remove your baby from the breast more easily by placing your little finger in his mouth, thus interrupting the vacuum produced by suction and facilitating the exit of the nipple from his mouth, without getting hurt. This apparent complex technique is nothing more than a necessary complement to something innate: your motherhood, and you should take it as good support for a process of adjustment and learning that necessarily takes time.

Premature incorporation of liquids or complementary feeding may produce a decrease in dairy production. As a result, the baby has a lower ingesta of energy and nutrients.

How to find out when your baby is hungry

It is essential to incorporate the concept that not always the fact that the baby cries mean that he is hungry or in pain. Every time your baby cries, you should investigate other causes that may justify the crying, such as being very warm, being cold, wet or dirty, needing to be talked to having excessive environmental noise. As you will notice, in this time of life the crying is a way to communicate for the baby.

If after reviewing all the causes that could be causing your baby's crying, you don't find any, hold him into your arms and give him his favorite pacifier. You will be surprised to see how quickly it calms down: what he needed was to be at ease in your arms. What a lucky baby he is to have his mother to hold him! Holding the baby when he needs it is not bad; on the contrary, it helps him to acquire greater security. People say that if you hold your baby a lot of time, he will be spoiled. I do not agree! The more you keep holding him when he needs it, the faster he will incorporate this security. Then, he will claim the arms only at the most important moments. Now, the baby may keep crying, while he is in your arms and with his pacifier. If it's been more than two hours since the last breastfeed, what's happening is that your baby is hungry. Do not delay his feeding more; place it to your breast.

The pacifier should be the one that the baby likes the most. You will have to change several of different models and forms until you find the one that satisfies your baby. Remember that he does not know how to hold it in his mouth, the strong mechanism of protrusion (bringing the tongue out) that allows him to suck the breast, will make the pacifier fall, giving the feeling that he rejects it. Place the baby in a position to suckle and allow the pacifier to bounce against your body; Over time he will learn to hold it.

Having a quiet and pleasant space is essential to establish that link and that unique communication that occurs between the mother and the baby at the time of breastfeeding. If your baby is restless, an environment with sufficient light is advisable so that he can see your face and stay "anchored" in your eyes while breastfeeding. During the first days, it is desirable to feed him lying down, and then to search for the position that allows you to be more comfortable to support your baby safely. A high backrest chair will facilitate the relaxation of your muscles avoiding contractures that generate pain at the end of the feeding. You can add if you need it, a small stool to support the feet, helping to support your baby better.

To have, a good production of milk.

Taking care of yourself is the key to achieving good milk production. If you stay relaxed, eat well and drink enough fluids, you will have plenty of milk for your baby.

Rest as much as you can, particularly during the first weeks, and try to sleep a lot. Remember, when the baby sleeps, the mother sleeps.

Most of the milk is produced in the morning, or when you are more rested. If you get tense, the supply may be lower.

Leave aside the tasks of the house, doing only those that are necessary. In this way, you can pay more attention to your baby, and at the same time, you will feel more relaxed.

Make a varied diet, balanced, rich in healthy fats and protein. Avoid excess of carbohydrates.

Ask your doctor about vitamin supplements.

Drink plenty of fluids during the day. Allow thirst to be the guide of how much you need.

Squeeze all the milk the baby has not taken in the first feed of the day to stimulate the breasts to continue producing milk.

Some foods can change the taste of milk; It is not bad as the baby gets used to receiving foods with different flavors. In this way, he will prepare himself to accept a rich, healthy and complete diet.

Positions to breastfeed

Lying down is the ideal position to feed the baby at night: if it is too small, it may be necessary to give some support with a pillow. This position will be pleasant if you find it uncomfortable to sit down. If you have had a Caesarean section and you are still sore, try to lie down with the baby's feet under your arm.

Lying position: it is a comfortable alternative and keeps a restless baby away from the tender incision of a cesarean section.

Seated position: make sure you have your arms and back supported and that you are relaxed. Make sure the baby has a free hand to touch and caress your body.

With the baby's legs under the mother's arm: this position allows the baby to extract milk from the ducts that are in the axillary area of the mammary gland. In this way, you can prevent the accumulation of milk in this sector, causing pain and discomfort or, what is worse, the formation of hardness resulting in mastitis. Try to use this position at least twice a day in the first weeks of the child's life.

The first feeds of the newborn: sit comfortably in an upright position with your back supported, ideally in a low chair without armrests, or in bed with many pillows behind the back. If it gives you confidence, place a pillow on your legs to place the baby at the right height, or raise a knee to support your body. **Do not bend your back when leaning forward.**

When the baby is some weeks old: once you are both experts, you will discover that any relaxed posture is good. The position of sitting on the bed or the floor with crossed legs is excellent, especially if you can rest your back on pillows or a piece of furniture.

Sitting comfortably: it can take up to an hour to finish; inspire deeply and relax the shoulders. The more relaxed you are, the easier it will be for your baby. Give him the most natural contact with your skin. If you are in private, undress your chest, and you will see how, without clothes in between, its "grabs" better, that is, it leans on the chest properly and sucks effectively.

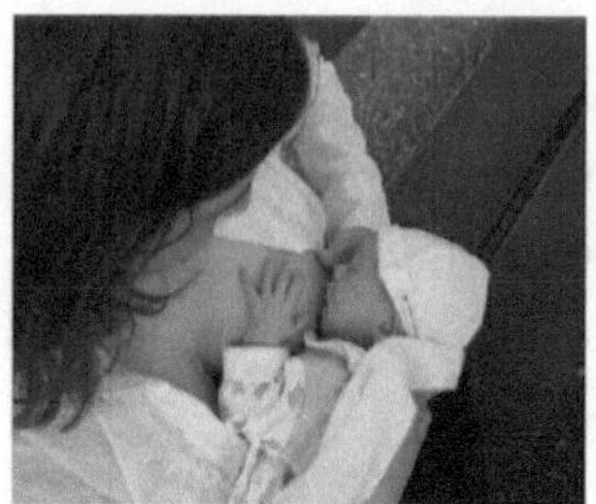

How to breastfeed twins?

A mother who achieved an adequate weight gain during pregnancy can breastfeed both babies. Your milk production will adapt to the suction, and you can offer the breast to the two together or separately. A comfortable position for both of them to breastfeed is sitting on the bed, surrounded by cushions where you can place the baby comfortably. Your partner can help you make sure you are comfortable, being on hand to lift and change babies, especially if one feeds faster than the other. If they suck in simultaneously, they will stimulate more milk production and allow you to have a longer time of rest. If you have been separated from babies for a while, in the beginning, because they were born prematurely, feeding them to the breast will allow you to know them and enjoy their proximity.

Feeding twins - especially when they are very small and eat little milk each time and need to feed often - will take a long time, so the first days you can feel very tired. 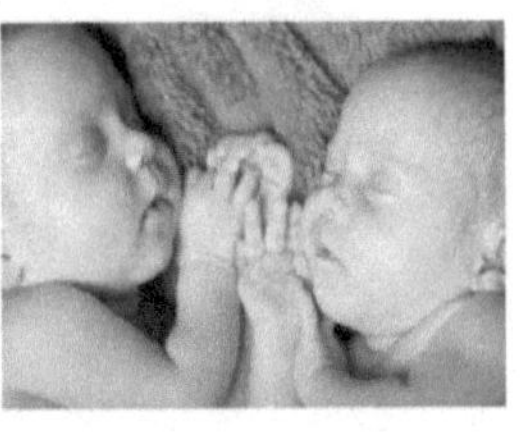
It is necessary to request all possible support and help (husband, family and friends) to establish a routine in the diet and acquire the skills necessary to care for two babies. If the pediatrician found that breastfeeding is not enough for both, one possibility is to feed one of the babies with the breast, while the other receives milk with formula and in the next feeding, feed them in reverse. Another option is to breastfeed the two of them at the same time and then offer them a bottle of formula.

Special Bras

It is essential always to wear a bra that holds your breasts well when you breastfeed. You should try it before buying it and look for ones with openings in front and with wide straps that do not hurt your shoulders. Quick-opening bras are ideal for opening with one hand while holding the baby with the other. A good bra will reduce the discomfort in case the breasts are inflamed. The aerating shells are very useful to keep the breasts dry, avoiding in this way that they get hurt by being very wet.

How to breastfeed correctly?

Milk is produced in glands that are beyond the fatty tissue, so the size of the breast is not indicative of the amount of milk that the mother will produce. Milk is produced about the quantity extracted and the demand of the baby. A more than enough supply of milk is generated in the mother's breast for each feeding. That is why moms should not worry that they will run out of milk if the baby is fed regularly. On the contrary, the breasts are stimulated to produce by the same reflex act of suction of the baby, so that the more you suck, the more milk will be produced. During the lactation period, the amount of milk available will vary according to the needs of the baby, and, once the baby begins to ingest solids, milk production will decrease.

For this reason, it is important not to incorporate any liquid or porridge before six months of age. At first, the baby will feed little and often. Around two months, will begin to feed every four hours and will take more milk than before in each shot. Regarding the time you keep the baby in each breast, it can be said that this depends on the interest he shows in sucking.

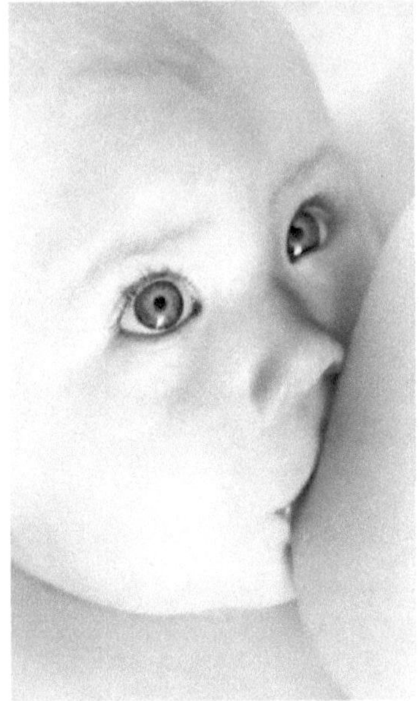

If the baby continues to breastfeed once your breast is empty, he may do so because he enjoys the sensation. It is not wrong for him to do this as long as it does not hurt or inflame your breasts. Breastfeeding creates a strong bond between mother and child if it is done in a pleasant and relaxed environment. It is important that the baby sees the mother and that she smiles and talks while breastfeeding. The child associates the pleasure of feeding with the sight of this face, the sound of this voice and the smell of this skin. The baby should be encouraged to look at the breast by gently stroking the nearest cheek. By doing it, you will help him develop the peri oral reflex, and he will immediately turn to the breast with his mouth open.

Possible problems during breastfeeding

Some difficulties usually appear at the beginning of this complex and new task for the mother. However, it is not a reason to be alerted. It is important to understand that, like mothers, children are also going through a period of learning, in which both will need time to adapt to each other. It is usual for the newborn, during the first 24 to 36 hours, not to breastfeed too much or too hard. But if this extends longer, it is possible that there is some drawback. One of the most common disadvantages is the difficulty of breathing caused by suckling. It is possible that the breasts cover the fins of the nose. In this case, the feeding nurse should gently hold the breast back, just above the areola, to move it away from the baby's face.

Another possible option is that the baby has a stuffy nose or difficulty breathing, in this case, it is essential to go to the pediatrician to evaluate what to do; The problem is usually solved with a nasal aspirator to remove the snot or snuff in the nose.

A different possibility is that the child is restless. A baby who has cried because of hunger is too tense to breastfeed. At this point, the interaction between mom and baby becomes more important. It is she who will reassure him: singing, caressing him, talking to him or simply holding him firmly.

In the specific case of premature babies, the role of the mother becomes even more important; She must be persistent and patient since the baby will have a harder time breastfeeding. In very few opportunities should be considered the option of giving supplementary bottles that can encourage the baby to stop breastfeeding. Most babies enjoy breast sucking a lot, just as moms feel a lot of pleasure while their baby is breastfeeding. In the case of premature babies, it is necessary to wake them up to feed them with some regularity, since as being so small they tend to fall asleep and skip a breastfeed.

Another difficulty may arise at the time of breastfeeding if the baby is not relaxed or satisfied. The problem here may be that the baby is not well attached to the breast and does not get enough milk. It is always important to verify that you place the child in the correct position.

Special cares

The hygiene of the breasts and nipples is very important; they should be cleaned daily and carefully with water. The use of toilet soap is not recommended since it dries the skin and can cause cracked or sensitive nipples. It is important to dry them both after routine hygiene and after breastfeeding the baby. Milk leaks are very common, in which case you may use discs or absorbent cloths.

If the nipples are cracked, it is necessary to treat them properly and immediately as they can get worse and crack more. In this case, the mother should feed the baby only with that breast that is not hurt and wait until the other is cured. One possibility may be to extract the milk manually and give it with a bottle or teaspoons. Specifically, in the case of cracks, a series of precautions can be taken to prevent them: to ensure that the baby introduces both the nipple and the areola when suckling, gently move the baby away from the breast once it has finished feeding and keep the nipples always dry.

Sometimes, it usually happens, towards the end of the first week, before regularizing breastfeeding, that the breasts are sore, congested and quite hard to the touch. The baby will find it more difficult to suck directly from the nipple, so it will be necessary to extract some milk before feeding it to relieve congestion. It is also advisable to use an appropriate bra to reduce pain.

Another fact to consider is the possible obstruction in some duct, which causes the inflammation of the breast, known as mastitis. It usually occurs after cracking or obstruction of an over infected lactiferous duct, being stress and fatigue contributing factors. It is essential not to stop breastfeeding, to rest, to drink fluids in response to thirst, to offer the child the compromised breast, to breastfeed and to empty frequently with proper position and breast placement; use extraction techniques, antibiotics, and anti-inflammatories.

Mastitis is recognized because the breast acquires signs of inflammation. Be careful because if you do not take it seriously and you do not treat it, mastitis can lead to a breast abscess. In this case, the mother will have all the symptoms mentioned and fever.

During the period of lactation, your body will require a greater supply of energy. It is not advisable to perform any low-calorie diet, nor to perform strenuous exercises. Having a varied and healthy diet is necessary. Surely you will be thirstier, so you will drink more liquid.

It is perfectly possible to maintain exclusive breastfeeding on returning to work.

There is no evidence to indicate that you should avoid any particular food. Foods or drinks high in caffeine (tea, coffee, mate, chocolate, cola drinks, among others) should be consumed in moderation. It is important that the mother does not smoke because it decreases milk production, and that she does not take any medication during the period of lactation since they can pass into breast milk and affect the baby. It is advisable to consult the doctor if you have any questions.

Breastfeeding and work

One of the biggest concerns for the mother who is breastfeeding is to think that at some point she will have to return to work. Also, it is very likely to ask: "Can I continue breastfeeding?", "Is it better not to breastfeed if you do not get used to the bottle later?", "Can I get milk at work? ", etc. Before all these questions there is only one answer:

You will have to prepare yourself a month after delivery and talk with the pediatrician about your return to work, what your plans are, your work schedule, distance, and who will take care of the baby. If you cannot take it to work or have it close to breastfeed, you should start as soon as possible to practice the extraction of milk to develop it with a certain degree of expertise.

You will have to extract milk once or twice a day after the breastfeeding's and kept it in well-closed and labeled sterile bags or jars, write down the date and store it in the freezer. These shots (60 cc is ideal) may be used; for example, someday you return a little later than planned or if the amount reserved for the baby is not enough when you are working. It is frequent for women to get enough milk during work or between breastfeeds, enough for two intakes. Milk extraction should be done in a quiet place and a comfortable position. You can stimulate the milk drop thinking about the baby or looking at a picture of him. The use of the breast pump is a fundamental aid. It is necessary to empty the entire breast and not exceed ten minutes of extraction in each one. The milk can be kept in the refrigerator and taken home for next day use.

Milk can be preserved:

• At room temperature: 12 hours.

• At 75° F (25 °C): 4-6 hours.

• In the refrigerator: 3-5 days.

• In the freezer of the refrigerator: 14 days.

• In the freezer: 3-4 months.

A way to preserve the milk components, consists on warm the bottle by submerging it in a container with hot water. It should never be heated by direct fire or microwave. Please, discard any milk.

It is important that if you work and breastfeed, you can have the chance to rest enough and have peace and family support to achieve it.

From birth to six months attention is focused on three main functions: suction, breathing and swallowing. In the process of breastfeeding important muscular functions are performed, and the child synchronizes his breathing with muscular activity. The movements of the muscles of the tongue, lips, and cheeks provide the necessary stimuli for the harmony of the face and the subsequent development of the jaws and teeth. At the time of birth all the milk teeth have already been formed but the development of the roots, which keep the tooth in its basket of the maxillary bone, has not yet begun.

The development of the teeth follows a strict order, but deviations from the parameters calculated for the general population should not be considered abnormal. Some children have an early rash, and their first tooth appears at four months or, on the contrary, they have a delayed rash, and they arrive at 14 months without any visible tooth in the mouth; then this delay is neutralized, and normally the first dentition is completed around the third month of life. Dental eruption is a physiological process. The milk teeth can erupt without producing symptoms, however in many infant's redness and swelling of the mucosa covering the tooth is observed. During this period the baby may show signs of local irritation and tends to rub the gum with his fingers or with some object, which causes drooling. An inflammatory reaction occurs that can cause local reactions. The general symptoms are irritability, fever, lack of appetite, respiratory infections, diarrhea, constipation, hypersalivation, and rashes. There is controversy about whether the dentition can produce any of these symptoms or if they are simultaneous and independent. But we must conclude that there is no absolute association, although local inflammation can cause irritability.

BOTTLE FEEDING

If for some reason you could not breastfeed your child, you will also grow healthy and strong receiving formula milk. These kinds of milk have been modified over time and present characteristics similar to breast milk, but because they don't come from mother's milk, they lack the immunological components of it. The fact of not being able to breastfeed or not wanting to do it does not imply you are a better or worse mother.

Establishing a good emotional bond is essential for the development of the baby. Babies who are fed with bottle do not need special care but should promote greater physical contact, unlike the small ones who are breastfed, to promote and strengthen the bond between the baby and the mother.

At first, it can be a bit complicated, but once you get used to sterilizing and preparing the bottles, everything will seem easy and simple. It is important that you have at least eight bottles so that you can prepare all your children's needs only once a day and keep them ready for him when he demands them. Prepare them at once and keep them in the refrigerator.

There are two sizes of bottles, some for very young babies and others for those who need to take more milk. There is a wide variety of brands of liquid or powdered artificial milk, bottles, and teats that allow food to be increasingly simple for mothers who for one reason or another have had to resort to the bottle to feed your son.

Colostrum cannot be replaced (the first food that the mother produces, and which is an indisputable source of defenses). For this reason, it is essential that you feed your newborn baby at least during the first days and, if possible, during the first month.

An advantage of bottle feeding is that the father can also participate, letting him build a loving and caring bond with the baby during the feeding process. It is important that you start doing it from the beginning so that you can feel more secure and get used to the technique and learning that requires feeding the baby.

How to choose the most suitable formula milk

There is a wide variety of milk brands for babies, and all of them must meet certain standards that regulate their manufacture. In all cases, attempts are made to resemble breast milk as much as possible. Some came in powder or are ready to use. The latter are presented in cans, cartons or bottles already prepared packaged by the UHT system (sterilization at high temperature). Liquid formulas are more expensive than powdered milk; however, they are more convenient and practical.

In the case of milk powder, it is important that you follow the indications of preparation that each milk has correctly.

Consider that If you add a larger amount of powder than the one indicated in the instructions, the child will receive too many proteins and fats and little water, while, if you add a smaller amount, the baby will not be able to incorporate enough nutrients to grow healthily.

Required equipment

- Breast and lids
- Teats
- Funnel
- Measuring spoon Plastic tweezers to remove each element
- Plastic container to store the sterilized items

The use of the measuring spoon included in the milk container allows measuring the adequate amount of powder necessary for the preparation (try to keep it outside the container). You can use the back of a knife to level each scoop and make sure you are placing the exact amount. It is important that you do not squeeze the powder into the spoon.

Place the right amount of milk powder in the mix or bottle in case you prepare one, with the water boiled and cooled but still a little hot. You can use a funnel to help you fill your bottles. Shake the mixture of milk powder and water well until no lumps or residues remain. Then, you must place the sterilized teats face up in the bottles, with the lid that protects them, and you must keep them in the refrigerator at the top (to prevent food that can drip contaminating them).

Cleaning and preparation of bottles

When you prepare this type of milk, it is important to maintain proper hygiene. This warning is because milk is an ideal medium for the development of germs that cause intestinal disorders so that both bottles and teats, teaspoons, jars and lids should be washed and sterilized correctly.

You can find Sterilization equipment that may be useful in large stores and pharmacies. Most of them have a capacity of four to six bottles.

As the baby feeds at least seven to eight times throughout the day, all utensils should be sterilized twice daily, in the morning and at night. This process will vary over time as the baby begins to incorporate food and do not need to depend on so many bottles.

The most common way to sterilize is by boiling all the elements that are in contact with the milk and the baby, but you can also use a container with cold water and a chemical sterilant. For this method, equipment consisting of a plastic container and a tray where you can dip utensils may be necessary.

How to do it, step by step

The first step when preparing a bottle is to wash them, including teats, with soapy water, using a brush to remove all the remaining milk. Then they should be rinsed with running water. To clean the teats, you can use coarse salt to remove the adhering milk.

Then, the sterilizing unit or container should be filled with cold water until the corresponding signal and dissolve the number of sterilizing tablets that correspond according to the indications of each product. You should wait until they are completely dissolved to start introducing the bottles, teats, spoon, meter and all the equipment used. You must leave it the indicated time and when it is time to use it you should rinse it with boiled water and drain it. Take special care so that no air bubbles remain as this would prevent the correct sterilization of some parts.

If you decide to use the method of sterilization by boiling it is enough to put the elements in water, taking the precaution that they are completely submerged, and boil them for approximately thirty minutes. It can also be done in steam sterilizing units, as well as in special containers adapted to the microwave. The containers should be washed and boiled for at least thirty minutes, taking care to boil the teats separately and in a closed container.

It's time for the bottle!

When feeding your baby with a bottle, you must consider some essential points. You should wash your hands with soap and water before starting. In case you use powdered milk, the mixture must be prepared properly following the indications of each brand to the letter. In this way, the baby will receive the correct amounts of both nutrients and water. You can prepare several at a time and keep them in the refrigerator or as they are needed.

How to give it

First of all, you have to be in a comfortable and relaxed place, supporting your arms well and holding the baby half seated with his head on his bent elbow and his back along the forearm, which will allow him to swallow without problems.

Before giving the bottle, it is important to check the temperature and the flow of the milk. Gently caress your baby's cheek to stimulate the search reflex, then gently insert the teat into his mouth.

The suction reflex will help the child to take his food. If the baby has difficulty sucking the milk, the bottle should be gently removed to allow air to enter and then continue as before. The bottle should be positioned at an angle so that the baby does not swallow air with the milk.

Take special care that the shots are pleasant moments. It is important to talk, smile, sing so that the baby has a good association with the time of eating and establish a good bond with the mother or father. We must try to be in a quiet environment so that the baby receives his food relaxed and serene.

Babies who don't breastfeed usually do so less often than those who drink breast milk. They can eat regularly every three or four hours, taking around six to eight bottles a day, approximately 100 milliliters each. However, as time passes the shots will be less frequent and larger. It is important not to get carried away by the clock, but to allow the baby to determine when and how hungry he is.

It is not necessary to empty the bottle in every shot since if your baby eats without being hungry what we will achieve is that he vomits or eats in excess leading to more weight than expected.

Using too much can make your baby constipated and may also cause dehydration. If, on the other hand, the baby is left hungry, you may need to increase the ration (you should ask your doctor if this is the case). Please, discard the milk remains.

Be careful not to leave the baby alone leaning somewhere while taking the bottle. It is a dangerous habit because you can drown very easily. Also, you should not put him to bed at the time of giving him the bottle because the milk can accumulate in the back of the mouth and choke or, in the worst case, can suck the contents.

Night shots

During the night the baby will also need a shot at least once, and this probably contributes to your feeling of tiredness and tension. You have to rest as much time as possible, both day and night, and try to derive some tasks from the father.

At first, the baby will need to feed every four hours, but once you have reached five kilos, it is important to extend the time between shots until you get about six hours of uninterrupted night sleep.

Then, even though the baby has his routine, you must try to ensure that his last shot coincides with the time when the parents go to bed. This way you will not need to interrupt your sleep. If beyond all effort the baby keeps waking up and demanding a shot at dawn, you must be patient and wait until you do not need it anymore.

When they burp and regurgitate

When a baby burps, he eliminates and removes all the air that has swallowed at the time of taking the bottle. Swallowing air is more common in those children who use the bottle. However, the mother can prevent it by tilting the bottle so that the teat is always full of milk and not air.

If your baby swallows air while bottle feeding, they may feel uncomfortable and cry, if this is the case, hold your baby upright against your shoulder or propped forward on your lap, after the feed. Gently rub their back so any trapped air can find its way out. There's no need to overdo it – wind isn't as big a problem as many people think.

Another factor to consider is whether the baby tends to regurgitate the milk after each feeding. The most important cause of this problem is the excess of food, and therefore you should never insist that the baby finish his bottle. If the baby tends to vomit after the shots, it is important that you consult your pediatrician.

Tips for taking into account

- Set a time and a place to give your baby the bottle with ease.
- Test the temperature of the milk by dropping a few drops on your wrist: it should be warm rather than hot.
- The milk should come out drop by drop through the hole in the teat. If this does not happen, it is because it is too small, and the baby will get tired of sucking before being satisfied. You may enlarge it with a sterilized needle (you can do it by heating the needle to the point it is red). In some bottles, the flow can be regulated giving pressure to the thread. If, on the contrary, the hole was too big, the baby would receive a lot of milk in a short time, and it could choke; in this case, you need to change it.
- If at the end of the intake there is a little milk left, you should discard it because it will spoil immediately with the baby's saliva.
- Some moms prefer to heat the bottle even though it is good at room temperature. If your choice is using the microwave to heat the bottle it is preferable to use glass containers, without forgetting to shake the bottle - the microwave does not heat evenly - and control the temperature after that.
- Bottles can also be heated in a container with hot water placing them for a few minutes in a water bath or directly under the tap water while stirring.

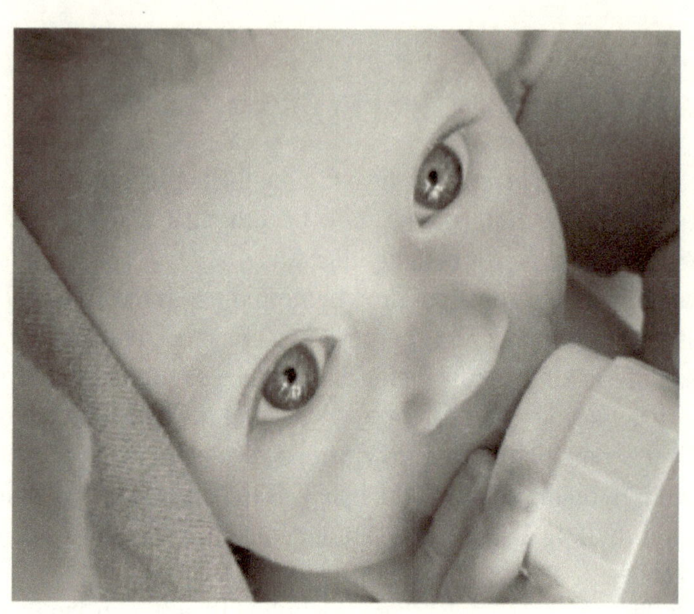

SAFETY FOR YOUR FAMILY

Safety is a major concern when it comes to feeding a child. Both food poisoning and choking can have serious consequences.

When you baby is about to start having solids, it is very important to stablish good habits concerning personal hygiene, and preparing, serving and storing food to prevent food poisoning. Infants and young children tend to have weaker immune systems than adults, which makes food poisoning very dangerous for this age group.

WASHING HANDS

WHEN TO WASH YOUR HANDS

- Before preparing food or feeding your baby
- After blowing your nose
- After going to the toilet
- After touching a pet
- After changing a nappy or checking your baby's nappy
- After contact with a sick child

HOW TO WASH YOUR HANDS

- Use soap and warm, running water.
- Rub hands to lather soap on backs of hands, under nails and between fingers for at least 10–15 seconds.
- Dry your hands thoroughly.
- Washing hands is the easiest and most effective way to stop the spread of disease.

TEACH YOUR CHILD TO WASH THEIR HANDS

- Have a step stool to help small children reach the sink.
- Have a hand washing song, to let them know it is time to wash their hands. Songs are a very useful tool to introduce habits to young kids, so be open to using them for toothbrushing time, bedtime, etc.
- Star to encourage children to rub and lather hands for at least 10–15 seconds.
- Set a good example by washing your hands together and talking about why it is important.

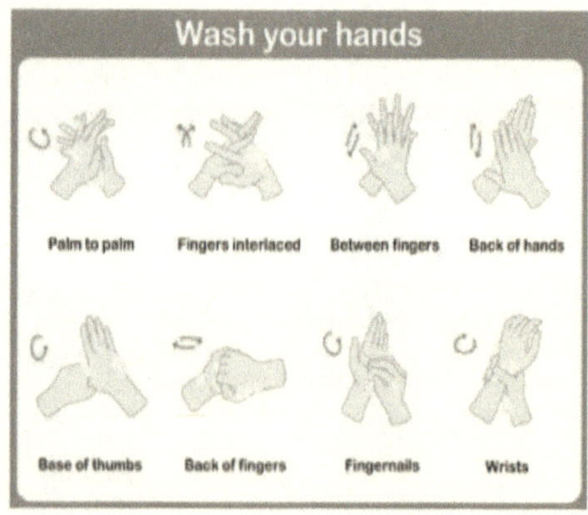

SAFE FOOD PREPARATION

Clean all food preparation areas, utensils and chopping boards with warm, soapy water before use, after preparing raw food and before contact with other foods.

If possible, use different utensils and chopping boards for raw foods and cooked foods.

Thaw frozen food in the refrigerator or rapidly in the microwave; do not leave on the bench to defrost. If thawing in the microwave the food must be cooked straight away.

Do not refreeze thawed foods.

Reheat foods quickly and thoroughly, so they are steaming.

Make sure poultry, mince, and sausages are cooked right through (no pink flesh or juices) before serving.

Keep fresh foods cold for preschool or while on outings by using an insulated lunch box and frozen drinks or ice pack.

SAFE STORAGE OF FOOD

- Bacteria that cause food poisoning can grow in foods such as meat, poultry, fish, eggs, milk or soy as well as rice, pasta, and vegetable dishes.
- Storing these foods in the refrigerator is important.
- Set your refrigerator at 40°F (5°C) or below.
- Store raw meat, fish and poultry in a container or plastic bag at the bottom of the refrigerator away from cooked and ready to eat foods.
- Cooked food should be rapidly cool by placing in the refrigerator as soon as it stops steaming.
- All food should be stored according to the directions on the container and should not be used after the expiry date.
- Don't eat food meant to be stored in the fridge if left out for more than two hours.

- Don't feed your baby directly form a container that is going to be stored for later. Dipping from spoon-to mouth and back to the container introduces bacteria for your baby into the rest of the food. This bacteria can continue to grow in the leftovers. So it is better to serve food into a separate dish and feed your baby from it. Please, throw away uneaten food from the dish.

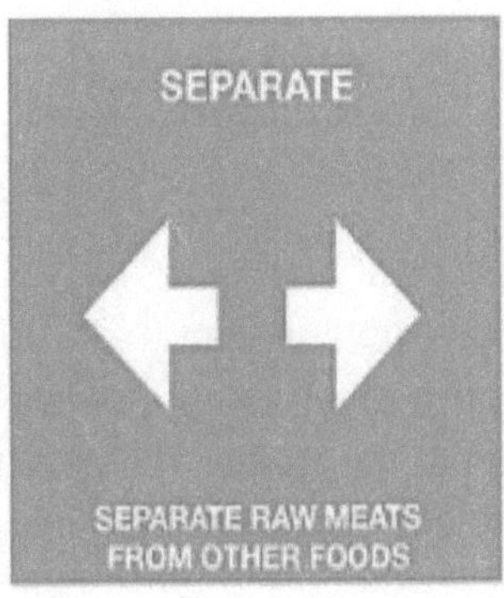

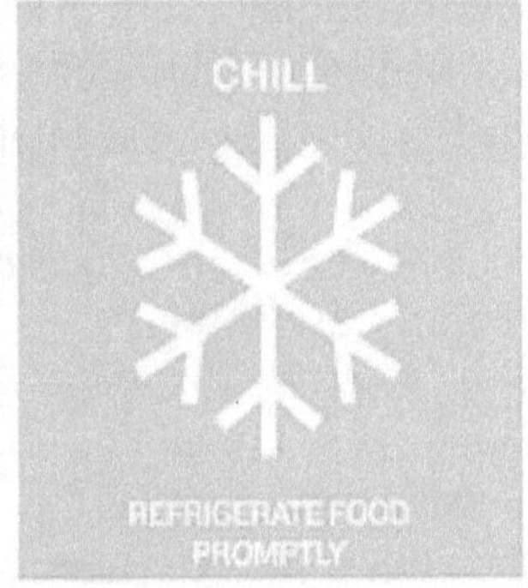

KEEP YOUR FAMILY SAFER FROM FOOD POISONING

How can I make eating safer for a child?

Choking is a common cause of injury, also leading to death in young children, because their small airways are easily obstructed. It takes time for babies to obtain and master the ability to chew and swallow food, and they may not be able to cough strongly enough to clear the obstruction.

Food is the most common cause of infant choking. However, small objects, parts from toys and certain types of behavior during eating — such as eating while distracted — also can cause infant choking.

So it is very important that you **always supervise young babies and children when they are eating.**

- Offer food in small amounts to prevent your baby from putting too much food in his mouths.
- Introduce foods in textures that are safe for your baby. Offer cooked foods before trying them raw. For example, try applesauce or well-cooked carrots first and then offer grated raw apples or carrots later.
- Cut food into small pieces until your child can chew and swallow food that is the texture of steak without coughing (around three years old usually)
- Do not give hard, crunchy foods to your child until he can consistently chew and swallow crusty bread without coughing. Hard, crunchy foods include hard candies, nuts, raw carrots, apples, fruit with pits, popcorn and sunflower seeds. Be aware that un-popped corn kernels are especially dangerous.
- Spread smooth peanut butter or other nut and seed butter thinly on crackers or bread. A chunk of nut or seed butter can form a "plug" that can block your child's airway.
- Make sure your baby is awake and alert before offering them food.
- Do not prop or leave a baby alone with a bottle. They could choke on the liquid.
- Have your baby sit up while eating and drinking.

- Do not give your child anything to eat or drink while he is walking, playing, or sitting in a moving car, bus or stroller.
- If your child is laughing or crying, settle them before offering them food. Have them sit down and eat in a calm, quiet environment.
- Teach your child to chew their food well. Sit down and eat with him. Be a positive role model – take small bites, chew food well, and eat slowly.
- Teach older children not to give food or small toys to younger children.

NEVER LEAVE YOUR BABY OR TODDLER UNATTENDED WHILE EATING.

KEEPING YOUR CHILD SAFE WHEN EATING

- Test the temperature of food before feeding your child.

- Make sure your child is sitting upright when eating.

- Encourage your child to eat slowly and chew food well.

- Do not force-feed your child or put food in their mouth if they are crying or not ready.

- Avoid giving a young child food that may cause them to choke such as whole nuts, hard or raw vegetables, popcorn or lollipops.

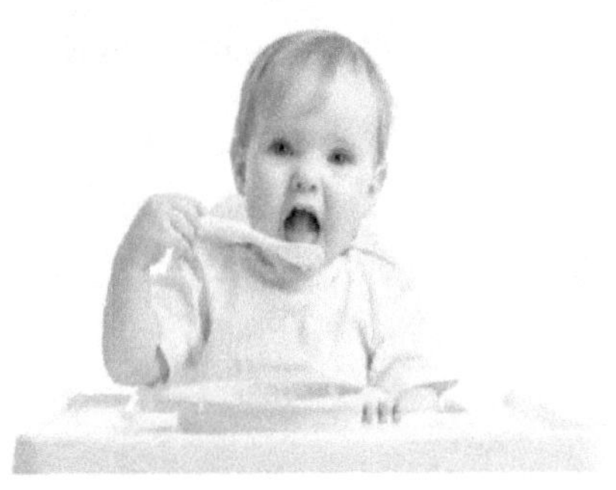

HOW MUCH FOOD?

You can use the amounts listed as a guide and ask your child's health care provider for additional help. At around six months, your baby can hold food in the palm, followed by the ability to hold food with the fingers.

AGE	FOOD	AMOUNTS PER DAY
Birth to 6 months	Breast / Milk Formula	18-32 ounces first three months
		28-45 ounces three to six months
6 Months	Breast / Milk Formula	28-45 ounces
	Infant Cereal/ Purees	4-8 tablespoons
6 to 9 Months	Plain Fruit Strained	3-4 tablespoons
	Yogurt unsweetened	1-2 tablespoons

	Vegetables Plain strained	3-4 tablespoons
	Meat Plain strained	1-2 tablespoons
	Iron-fortified Cereal	4-6 tablespoons
	Fruit juice unsweetened (delay orange, pineapple, grapefruit, and tomato juice)	2-4 ounces
	Breast / Milk Formula	24-32 ounces
9 to 12 Months	Iron-fortified Cereal	4-6 tablespoons
	Fruit juice unsweetened	4 ounces
	Vegetables	6-8 tablespoons
	Fruit	6-8 tablespoons
	Meat, fish, Poultry, egg yolk, yogurt.	4-6 tablespoons
	Crackers, toast unsweetened	½ - 1-ounce small portion

	Breast / Milk Formula	24-32 ounces

Portions are small in the first year. Not only are babies' stomachs very small, but it is important to remember that in the first year of life, most of their nutrients still come from their milk feeding.

Food Consistency by Age

Age	Food Form
Birth–4 months	liquid
4–6 months	strained
6–8 months	strained to mashed
8–10 months	mashed to minced
10–12 months	minced to chopped
12–36 months	chopped table food

CHAPTER 2: FIRST FOODS

(6 Months).

Introducing your baby to solid foods, sometimes called complementary feeding or weaning, should start when your baby is around six months old.

In the beginning, how much your baby eats is less important than getting them used to the idea of eating. They'll still be getting most of their energy and nutrients from breast milk or first infant formula.

Giving your baby a variety of foods, alongside breast or formula milk, from around six months of age will help set your child up for a lifetime of healthier eating.

Gradually, you'll be able to increase the amount and variety of food your baby eats until they can eat the same foods as the rest of the family, in smaller portions.

Babies first foods can be prepared easily, and they are cheap and healthy. These first foods should at first be mashed and smooth, but you can quickly move on to coarsely mashed foods and coarser textures.

You should start with a single food rather than a mixture.

Remember that your baby may only take a spoonful at first, but this will increase with time and practice

The PPP rule is of big help here

- be **P**atient (baby may only take a spoonful at first),

- be **P**repared (babies usually make a mess when eating),
- be **P**erseverant (try again in a day or so if your baby refuses the first time).

The amounts of foods eaten by your baby and their interest in food may be a little different from day to day.

Relax, this is normal and shouldn't cause any problems or concerns if your baby is growing well. **Always keep in touch with your pediatrician.**

When is the baby ready for solids?

Some Clues that your baby is ready for solids:

- Baby has good head control and able to sit up with support.
- Watching and leaning forwards when food is around.
- Reaching out to grab food or spoons to put in their mouth
- Opening their mouth when food is offered.
- Milk is not enough to feed him or her.

Why not before?

Starting on solids much earlier may cause your baby to breastfeed less, causing your breast milk to dry up sooner. Starting too early may also lead to a diet that's low in protein, fat, and other nutrients.

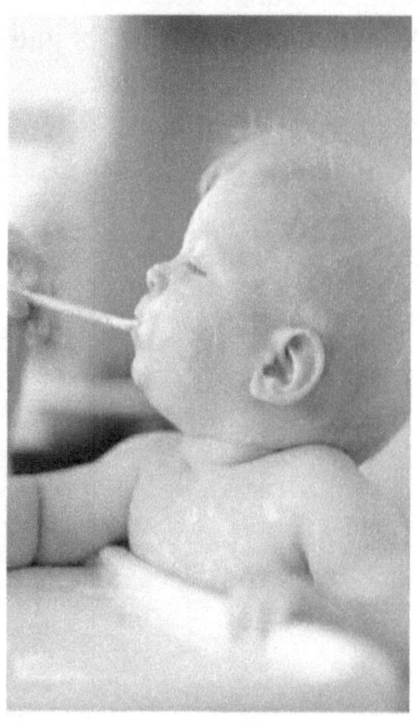

Babies that eat solids prematurely, who are not mature to do it, replace breastfeeding, and lose the value of this milk forever. By not being ready to eat solids, they gain almost none benefit from the new food, that takes a lot of time for them to digest

Solid food has more sodium and proteins that breast milk, and babies with less than six months of age, have immature kidneys that don't take well this overload. Also, the intestines have some enzymes that will grow since birth and will help to digest complementary food.

By the fifth or sixth month of age, baby start losing the suck reflex and Tongue thrust, and new vertical mouth movements appear that help babies to start chewing solids. Other problems on early introducing these foods are poor growing (because they stop taking breast milk) and diarrhea.

FOODS TO AVOID GIVING BABIES AND YOUNG CHILDREN

Salt

Babies shouldn't eat much salt, as it isn't good for their kidneys. Don't add salt to your baby's food or cooking water, and don't use stock cubes or gravy, as they're often high in salt.

Remember this when you're cooking for the family if you plan to give the same food to your baby.

Avoid salty foods like:

- bacon
- sausages
- chips with added salt
- crackers
- crisps
- ready meals
- takeaways

Sugar

Your baby doesn't need sugar. By avoiding sugary snacks and drinks (including natural fruit juice at the beginning and other fruit drinks), you'll help prevent tooth decay.

Saturated fat

Don't give your child too many foods that are high in saturated fat, such as crisps, biscuits, and cakes.

Checking the nutrition labels on foods can help you choose foods that are lower in saturated fat.

Honey

Occasionally, honey contains bacteria that can produce toxins in a baby's intestines, leading to infant botulism, which is a very serious illness. Don't give your child honey until they're over one year old. Honey is a sugar, so avoiding it will also help prevent tooth decay.

Whole nuts and peanuts

Whole nuts and peanuts shouldn't be given to children under five years old, as they can choke on them.

You can give your baby nuts and peanuts from around six months old, as long as they're crushed, ground or a smooth nut or peanut butter.

If there's a history of food allergies or other allergies in your family, talk to your GP or health visitor before introducing nuts and peanuts.

Some cheeses

Cheese can form part of a healthy, balanced diet for babies and young children, and provides calcium, protein, and vitamins.

Babies can eat pasteurized full-fat cheese from 6 months old, including hard cheeses, such as mild cheddar cheese, cottage cheese, and cream cheese.

Babies and young children shouldn't eat mold-ripened soft cheeses, such as brie or camembert, or ripened goats' milk cheese and soft blue-veined cheese, such as Roquefort, as there's a higher risk that these cheeses might carry a bacterium called listeria.

Many kinds of cheese are made from unpasteurized milk. It's better to avoid these because of the risk of listeria. Please, check labels on cheeses to make sure they're made from pasteurized milk.

But these cheeses can be used as part of a cooked recipe as listeria is killed by cooking. Baked Brie, for example, is a safer option.

Cow's milk

Feed only breast milk or infant formula to drink in the first year—no cow's milk until after one year.

Raw and lightly cooked eggs

Babies can have eggs from around six months. Eggs are in the top 8 of all allergens, but recommendations for introducing eggs to babies have been changing. It is the white of the egg that is allergenic and not the yolk.

Rice drinks

Rice Milk is low in fat which is not recommended for those under two years of age, and it is also low in (if not completely devoid of) protein. "It contains more carbohydrates as compared to cow's milk, but less protein and calcium and no cholesterol and lactose. It also may contain arsenic which is toxic for your baby.

Raw jelly cubes

Raw jelly cubes can be a choking hazard for babies and young children.

If you're making jelly from raw jelly cubes, make sure you always follow the manufacturers' instructions.

Raw shellfish

Raw or lightly cooked shellfish, such as mussels, clams, and oysters, can increase the risk of food poisoning, so it's best not to give it to babies.

Shark, swordfish, and marlin

Don't give your baby shark, swordfish or marlin. The amount of mercury in these fish can affect the development of a baby's nervous system.

Source: NHS Food

FOOD ALLERGIES

Approximately 6 to 8 percent of children under age four have a food allergy, and 4 percent of all adults do as well.

For kids with a family history of allergies or frequent rashes, you can postpone the introduction of certain foods. Be careful when introducing food that may cause allergies to your baby.

Be careful enough to Introduce one single-ingredient new food at a time, to make sure your baby is not allergic or intolerant to these foods.

The foods most likely to cause a food allergy are eggs, milk, wheat, soy, peanuts, tree nuts, fish, and shellfish.

Cow's milk is the most likely problem for food. Up to 7 percent of infants have trouble digesting milk proteins. Try not to give your baby cow's milk before he is 2 years old.

To Pin Down the problem, your doctor may suggest eliminating one food at a time.

An upset tummy, a rash, or a lack of weight gain may signal that your baby has a food intolerance or even an allergy.

There is a risk of allergies on babies, so be sure to know allergies from both parents' families and try to avoid these products…

Always seek advice from your doctor

Symptoms of food intolerances

- Most frequently a rash around their mouth or cheeks which might spread further
- runny or stuffed nose and red, itchy eyes
- increased spitting up
- Diarrhea

With the baby seated on his chair or your lap and his food plate in front, you will need to motivate and show what is going to happen.

You may (if needed) knock the spoon with the border of the plate to make a sound and catch his attention, when the baby focusses his attention on the spoon, only then place the spoon on his eye level and when he sees the food, take the spoon closer to his mouth.

Put the spoon between his lips and allow the baby to take the food, don't force it as it may give him nausea or even vomit.

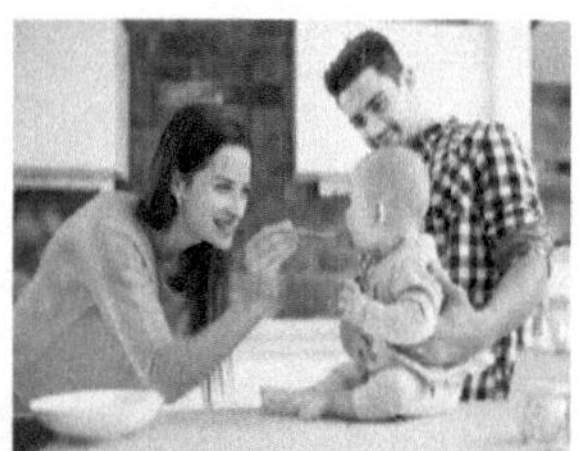

If the baby pushes the food out, grab it with the spoon again and try again.

Introducing solids to the baby may take several months until you can do it adequately and pleasingly, so no need to rush it.

Be ready for extreme messes. If the thought of having avocado spread all over your baby's highchair tray and in their hair makes you flinch, well, that's just the beginning. Babies make a lot of mess while eating, and that's all part of their learning process. Wash their hands before sitting down and let them have fun. It's all part of learning and building positive associations.

Try to be patient as your baby experiments and learns and be tolerant of messes. Your baby will likely enjoy playing with a spoon, but most of the food will fall off it. It's natural for your baby to "make a mess" while learning about food. Until your baby can handle a spoon better, you can give your baby a clean spoon to hold while you feed him or her with a different spoon.

To help reduce your clean-up, use a child's high chair that has a detachable tray and raised rims. The rims on the tray help keep dishes and food from sliding off. And you can carry the tray to the sink for cleaning. Cover the seat with a removable, washable pad. Also, think about covering the floor around the high chair.

Remember that your child is learning by experimenting.

APPLE PUREE

🐾 5-6 months

♠ 2 servings

Ingredients

1 Organic Apple (peeled, cored, diced)

Boiled Water (as needed if using a stove)

Directions (using a microwave)

1. Put the diced apple in a microwave bowl.

2. Cover with a plastic film and made some small cuts on the film to allow the steam to escape.

3. Cook 3 minutes at Maximum power(100%).

4. Leave it there for a minute to cool down

5. Take the film out and strain the fruit through a colander or process it.

6. Let it cool enough before giving it to the baby

Don't store this puree for more than 24 hours. If you want to do it store in the freezer.

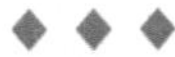

Directions (using a stove)

1. Put the diced apple saucepan

2. Add some water, enough to cover the bottom of the pan.

3. Cover the pan with a lid.

4. Cook for 6 minutes until the apple is soft.

5. Strain or process the apple and let it cool enough before giving it to the baby

PEAR PUREE

5-6 months

2 servings

Ingredients

1 organic Ripe Pear (peeled, cored, diced)

Boiled Water (as needed)

Directions

1. Put the diced, cored ripe pear in a small saucepan.

2. Add 2 tablespoons of water.

3. Cover with a lid and cook 3 to 5 minutes until the fruit is very soft.

4. Mash or process it

5. Let it cool down before serving.

BANANA PUREE

5-6 months

2 servings

Ingredients

1 Banana

Directions

1. Peel the banana, cut in the middle (long side) and remove the center.

2. Add 2 tablespoons of water. If the banana is ripped enough, you can mash it and serve immediately.

3. If not, you can cook it with a couple of water tablespoons and then mash it together with a fork. This way puree will be softer and more suitable for babies.

Prepare it just before eating, so you avoid banana oxidation.

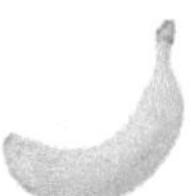

SWEET POTATO PUREE

🐢 5-6 months

🔔 4 servings

Ingredients

1 cup of organic sweet potato.

Directions

1. Boil the sweet potato in 1 or 2 cups of unsalted water (or roast it)

2. Mash it with a fork, add some boiled water to adjust the texture.

PEACH PUREE

🍼 5-6 months

🍽 2 servings

Ingredients

2 organic Ripe Peach (Washed, peeled, cored, diced)

Boiled Water (as needed to adjust consistency)

Directions

1. Puree peaches in a food processor or blender until smooth. Add water as needed to reach desired consistency.

Tips:

A ripe peach will give slight juice when you squeeze it.

Buy organic fruit. Try to eat seasonal fruits; peaches are available in summer.

You can Wash the peach with a mixture of three parts water and one part white vinegar to remove bacteria. Rinse under cool running water and dry.

Easy peeling of peaches: Bring water to a boil in a medium saucepan and then add peaches to the water for about 45 seconds. With a slotted spoon, remove peaches from boiling water and plunge into an ice bath immediately. After peach has been fully submerged, remove and peel the skin with your fingers or a sharp paring knife. It may help if your baby is constipated.

You can refrigerate leftover peach puree in BPA-free containers for up to 3 days. Freeze leftovers for up to 3 months.

BUTTERNUT SQUASH PUREE

🐢 5-6 months

♨ 4 servings

Ingredients

1 cup of organic butternut squash, washed seeds removed, peeled and chopped.

Boiled Water (as needed to adjust consistency)

Directions

1. Boil the butternut squash in 1 or 2 cups of unsalted water (or roast it)

2. Mash it with a fork, add some boiled water to adjust the texture and consistency.

Butternut squash is pure and simple, with a sweet, nutty flavor.

When roasted, it takes on a velvety texture.It's usually a child's favorite because of its sweeter taste.Butternut squash can be roasted at 425ºF until tender (about 40mins).

You Can replace the Butternut squash with pumpkin.

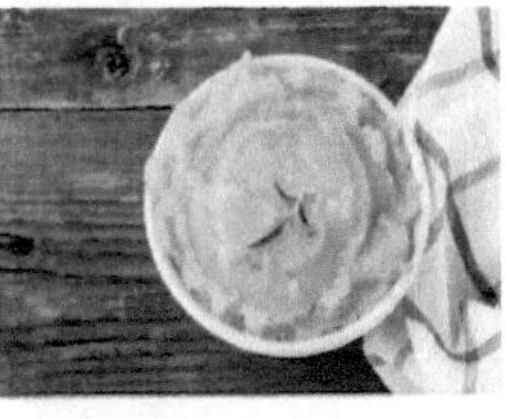

Like sweet potato puree, butternut squash puree is the ideal complement to a variety of other veggies, fruits, and meats.

Peak growing season is early fall through winter.

Look for butternut squash that is firm and free of cracks, bruises, or soft spots.

AVOCADO PUREE

🐛 5-6 months

🔔 4-5 servings

Ingredients

1 large ripe organic avocado

Directions

1. Slice avocado down the middle, lengthwise, working around the pit. Twist to separate each half until it pulls apart.

2. Score pit with a spoon. Twist the spoon to pull out the pit.

3. Scoop avocado meat out of its skin with a spoon and put it in a dish.

4. Use a fork to mash the avocado into a puree or use a blender or food processor to reach your desired consistency.

5. Add breastmilk, formula or water as needed to achieve the desired texture.

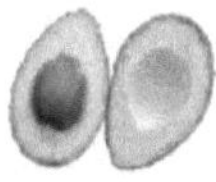

Omega-3-rich avocados are a great first introduction to solid foods. Avocados have a buttery, creamy texture that's easy for babies to mash between their gums.

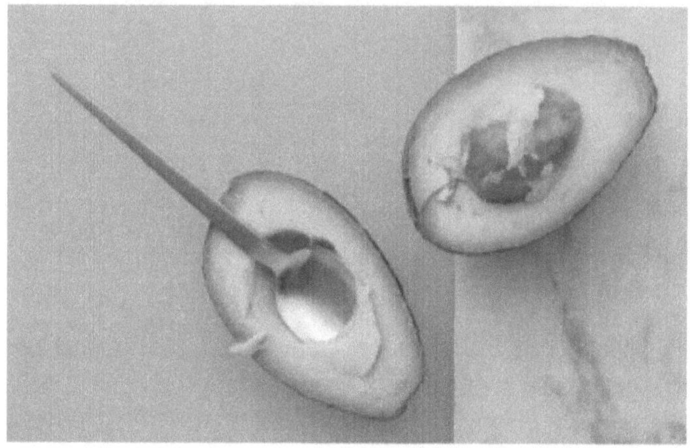

Store your batch of avocado baby food in an airtight container in the refrigerator for up to 72 hours.

PEAR AND RICE

This baby puree made from pears and rice cereal is a nutritious meal for your baby.

🐣 5-6 months

🍚 4 servings

Ingredients

1 organic pear (peeled, cored, diced)

3 oz (85g) of organic rice

Boiled Water (as needed)

Directions

1. Cook the rice in boiling water for 18 minutes

2. Strain it through a colander and mix it with the peeled and cored pear (be sure to take out all the seeds).
3. Add boiled water and process it till you get the desired consistency (creamy and soft).

Apple And Sweet Potatoes

Sweet potato is an ideal first food for your weaning baby due to its natural sweetness and smooth texture when blended.

5-6 months

4 servings

Ingredients

7 oz (200g) of organic Sweet Potatoes

3.5 oz (100g) of organic Apples.

Boiled Water (as needed)

Directions

1. Steam the sweet potato for about 10 minutes.

2. Add the apple (with no seeds) and steam for a further 5 minutes, until they are both soft.

3. In a food processor or blender, blend the sweet potato and apple, using as much water as necessary to reach the desired texture.

CHAPTER 3: INTRODUCING TEXTURES AND FLAVORS.

(6 to 9 Months).

This is one of the most influential periods in your baby's taste development. Your baby will most readily try and accept all kinds of foods at this age, so it's important to offer a variety of different flavors from meal to meal.

At this age, babies need to develop some new skills, such as chewing, dissolving in the mouth and swallow, to replace the suck reflex.

Usually, when kids discover this new skill, they enjoy this training very much.

By this age, kids should be able to sit straight on their chair and will start recognizing smells, textures, and flavors. They start differentiating things and using amazing faces with every new food introduced.

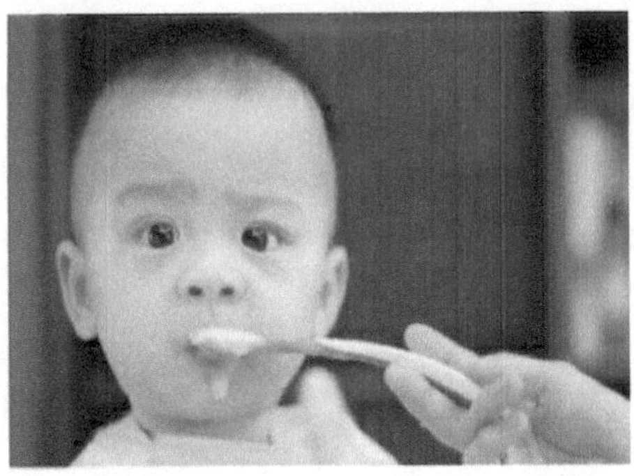

Eating solids at this age is mostly about offering your baby the opportunity to explore new flavors and textures. Breast milk or formula will remain your baby's primary nutrition source for the first year, so continue to give breast milk and formula just as you were before starting solids.

If you're breastfeeding, don't mix your breast milk with the purees for the first few attempts at eating. Until your baby shows that he really will eat it, most of the food will wind up somewhere else besides their stomach, like on the floor, their head, or the tray.

Your breast milk is too valuable to throw away, so mix the cereal, fruit or vegetable puree with a little water at first. When your infant is taking it well, then you can mix it with your breast milk.

At around six months old, offering a few tablespoons of food 1-3 times a day is enough. Start with thin, pureed foods, until your baby is comfortable with this texture. Next, move to lumpy, mashed foods, followed by finely chopped foods. First food sources are often cereal, mashed fruits, and veggies.

SOME NUTRITIONAL TIPS

The first six months of life, babies have enough nutrients reserves; after that, it's important that they start acquiring it from their meals.

CALCIUM

Calcium is important for bone and tooth health, blood clotting, neuron messaging, hormones, muscle contraction (including the heart!) and other processes. Good sources of calcium for your baby include breast milk, infant formula, yogurt; pureed leafy greens like kale, collard, and spinach, as well as pureed beans.

DHA

DHA is critical for brain growth and healthy development. It is an unsaturated omega three fat that can be found in oily fish (salmon, sardines, rainbow trout), Breast milk (if you include DHA rich foods in your diet), enriched infant formulas and other enriched foods.

IRON

Iron is a nutrient that's essential to your child's growth and development. Iron helps move oxygen from the lungs to the rest of the body and helps muscles store and use oxygen.

If your child's diet lacks iron, he or she might develop a condition called iron deficiency.

Iron deficiency in children can occur at many levels, from depleted iron stores to anemia — a condition in which blood lacks adequate healthy red blood cells. Untreated iron deficiency can affect a child's growth and development.

Babies are born with iron stored in their bodies, but a steady amount of additional iron is needed to fuel a child's rapid growth and development. Here's a guide to iron needs at different ages:

Age group	The recommended amount of iron a day
7 - 12 months	11 mg
1 - 3 years	7 mg
4 - 8 years	10 mg
9 - 13 years	8 mg

PROTEINS

Protein is an important component of our skin, hair, nails, muscles, blood, and bones. While most of us eat plenty of protein, it is important to offer protein-rich foods. Breast milk and formula are sources of protein for now, but for first foods, you can try pureed meat and poultry; yogurt; pureed beans, pureed tofu, and quinoa. When ready to advance textures, softly cooked flaky fish is a great protein source.

VITAMIN D

Babies need vitamin D for healthy growth and development. It helps them build strong, healthy bones and teeth. Babies who don't get enough vitamin D are said to have a deficiency. If the levels are low enough, they are at risk of getting rickets, a disease that affects the way bones grow and develop.

This vitamin helps calcium to be absorbed.

Vitamin D comes from different sources:

- **Sunlight:** Vitamin D is formed naturally when skin is exposed to sunlight (2 hours of sun a week for a baby with clothes).
- **Certain foods** like liver or tuna
- **Vitamin supplement**

Remember, while your baby is under one year it's all about introducing a variety of flavors and textures and keeping it fun!

THE IMPORTANCE OF ROUTINES

It's important to try to have a routine during the first months of the baby, where you respect the sleeping time, gaming time, etc.

You can choose the time to introduce the new foods either at noon or at night (if the baby is not tired). Keep that routine as much as possible until you can introduce a second meal to the baby.

Every baby and every family are different, so try feeding the baby at different times until you find the best time for everyone and try to stick to it.

You can start using Highchairs, so baby is next to the table, and its more comfortable to him and to the person who is giving him the food.

Compare Highchairs, check the safety, quality and possibilities each chair gives you.

In the beginning, try a not so straight chair with a safety belt, to avoid the baby falling down from it.

As we said in the previous chapter, be prepared for big messes. Your baby is learning to eat, and this experience has to be a good one. I will never be insistent enough with the PPPs

- be **P**atient (baby may only take a spoonful at first),
- be **P**repared (babies usually make a mess when eating),
- be **P**erseverant (try again in a day or so if your baby refuses the first time).
- And have lost of fun with your baby!

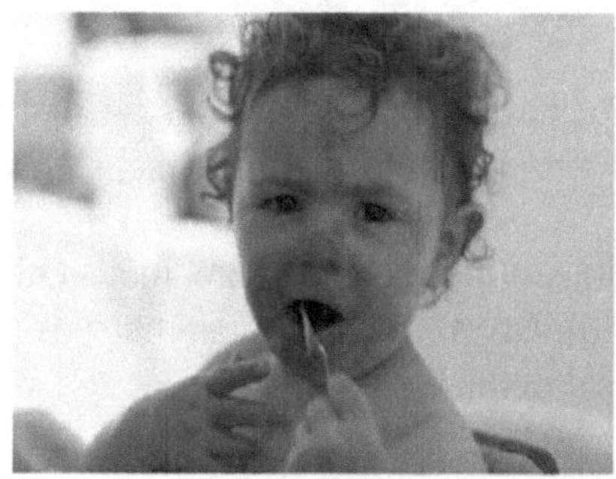

CALF LIVER WITH SMASH POTATOES AND PEAR

We recommend buying calf's liver when introducing liver to the baby. Calf's liver is particularly nutritious, with a good flavor. Please, try to buy livers from a local ecologic/organic shop to avoid the results of production methods that use daily supplemental hormones and antibiotics.

🍼 6-9 months

🍽 3-4 servings

Ingredients

¼ lb. (110g) Of calf liver.

1 egg yolk (organic if possible)

1 Large potato. 8oz (225g)

1 tbsp. oil

1 ripe pear 6.5oz (185g)

2 tablespoons of organic cereals (corn, rice, etc.)

Directions

1. Clean the liver and cook in a Teflon griddle or frypan, both sides for 8 minutes.

2. Cut as thin as possible

3. Cook an egg in water (starting with cold water) Count 10 mins since it started boiling, remove and let it cool down. **Use only the yolk**

4. Mash the yolk with a fork and mix with the liver.

5. Clean the pear, peel it and cook it in boiling water for 5 mins. Remove it from the fire and mash or process it.

6. Prepare a mashed potato by cooking them.

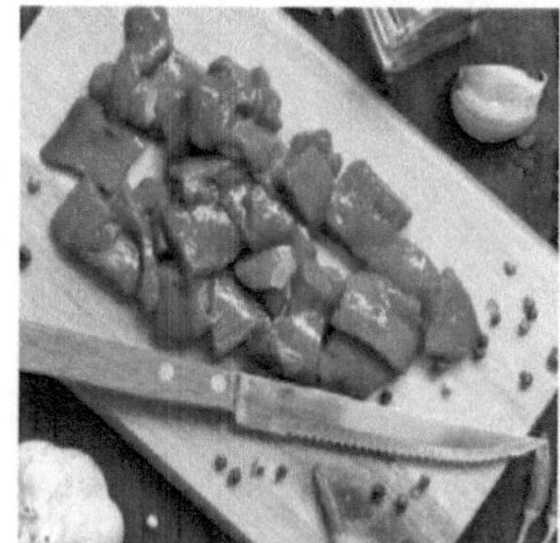

7. Mix the mash potatoes with the liver and pear, add some cereals and serve.

PINEAPPLE, SPINACH, AND PLAIN YOGURT PURÉE

🐢 +7 months

🍛 4-5 servings

Ingredients

1 cup (30 g) organic spinach leaves, packed.

1/2 pineapple outside cut off and chopped into chunks

1 cup of plain organic yogurt (250g)

Directions

1. Blend the spinach, pineapple, and yogurt in a blender until desired consistency is achieved.

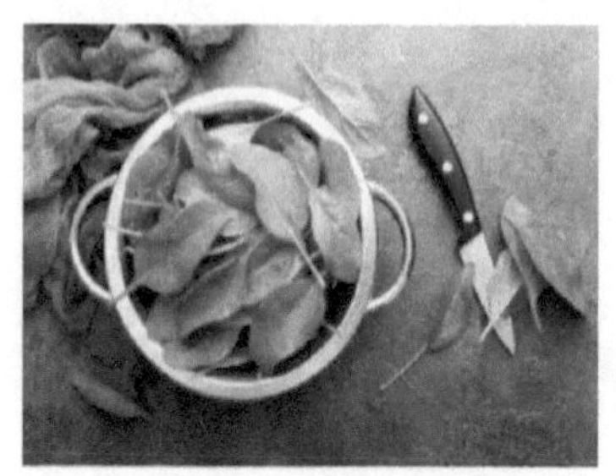

VITAMINS RICH PUREE

🍼 6-9 months

🍽 1-2 servings

Ingredients

½ Sweet Potato.

½ Carrot

½ Tomato

½ cup of sliced pumpkin or butternut squash

½ cup of formula milk

1 tsp. of oil.

Directions

1. Prepare a puree with the vegetables.

2. Add the tomato, processed without the skin and seeds.

3. Add the oil and milk and serve.

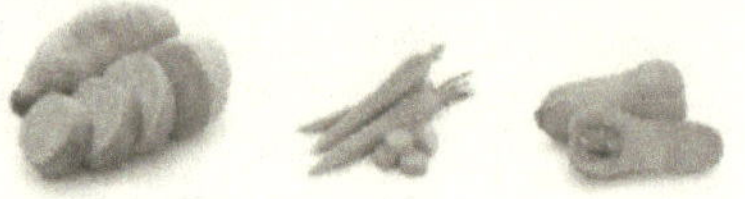

BANANA PUREE WITH BROCOLI AND SPINACH

🍼 6-9 months

🍽 2-4 servings

Ingredients

1 cup (70 g) chopped organic broccoli.

1 cup (30 g) organic spinach leaves, packed, stems removed

2 bananas peeled and sliced

Directions

1. Steam broccoli and spinach together for 3 to 5 minutes, until they are soft.

2. Reserve the water from the steamer.

3. Blend the mixture in a blender with the banana slices until puréed. Add
    1 teaspoon of reserved

water at a time, if necessary, until desired consistency is achieved.

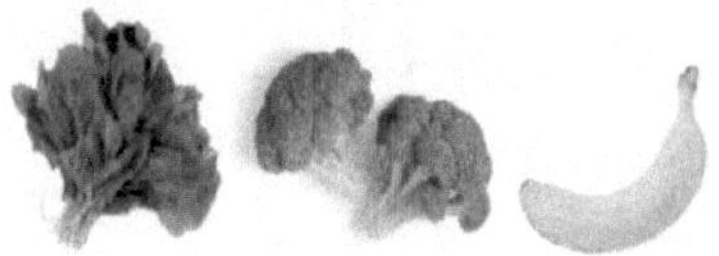

RASPBERRY PEAR PUREE

🐾 6-9 months

🍲 4-6 servings

Ingredients

2 organic pears peeled and steamed.

1/2 cup of organic ripe raspberries.

Directions

1. Just blend all the ingredients.

If your berries are not ripe enough, you can steam them a little.

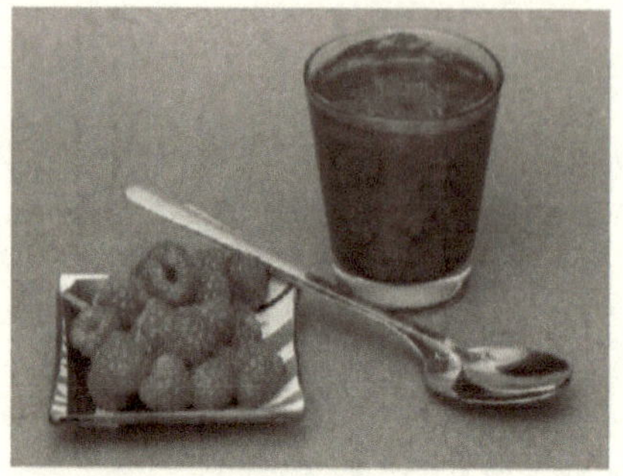

Berries can be a healthy part of your child's diet soon after she begins to eat solid food, usually when the baby is around 6-9 months old. But if your baby has chronic eczema or a food allergy, talk to the doctor first.

You can add some full-fat plain yogurt to this mix as well.

BABY PASTA WITH BROCCOLI CREAM

+8 months

2-3 servings

Ingredients

1 cup of baby pasta (like the Small stars or shells). Try to start with whole wheat organic pasta form the beginning.

1 cup of broccoli.

2 Tbsp. of heavy cream.

Directions

1. Cook the baby pasta in boiling water.

2. Strain it through a colander, cool it down with some water to avoid them to keep cooking.

3. Boil the broccoli for 6 minutes, strain and process it (or mash it with a fork).

4. Mix the cream, the baby pasta and the broccoli puree in a saucepan,

heat it, and serve. 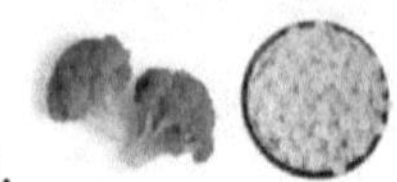

RED LENTILS AND CARROTS

6-9 months

2 servings

Ingredients

2 carrots.

1/2 cup of red lentils (100g).

1 tbsp. Oil.

Directions

1. Top and tail and peel the carrot, and slice up into 1cm slices

2. Rinse the red lentils then place in a saucepan with the carrots.

3. Boil the lentils with the carrots in water until both are tender.

4. Blend and add the oil.

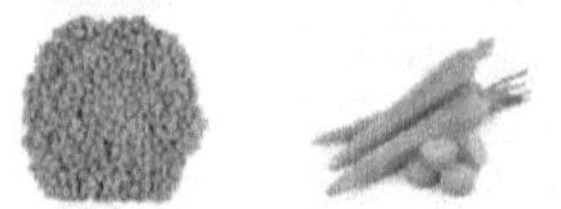

RED LENTILS AND SPINACH

🐢 6-9 months

🍽 3 servings

Ingredients

1/2 cup of spinach washed and steamed.

1/2 cup of red lentils (100g).

1 boiled water, breast milk or formula for consistency.

Directions

1. Boil the rinsed lentils until they are tender.

2. Prepare a puree with the boiled lentils and the steamed spinach.

3. Add water until you get the desired consistency.

4. Once you have ruled out a dairy allergy, you can add a teaspoon of parmesan cheese to add a little more flavor.

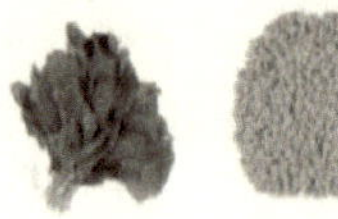

CHAPTER 4: BABY EATS BY HIMSELF.

(9 to 12 Months).

Your baby is getting bigger, independent and autonomous and acquiring new physical abilities that require more coordination and muscular strength. He can crawl, sit, maybe walk and roll, feeling happy and encouraged by the freedom he is acquiring little by little.

From 9 months solid foods start to be the basis of your baby's diet. He already wants to eat alone, he chews food better, and he is prepared to incorporate ground or chopped foods that have more texture than the puree he ate at first.

He can now eat three meals a day, and his diet is practically similar to that of the rest of the family. Although the milk intake was reduced over the months, it is important that he still drinks 500 ml of milk distributed throughout the day in different cups; It is a good time to start leaving the bottle.

When babies are close to their first year, they love to experience with more tastes and foods, changing breast milk by solid food.

Each time he will need less help at mealtime. He may be impatient and want to grab the spoon so that he can feed by himself, but he still does not have enough coordination to do it. As it is still difficult for him to eat alone, you can implement the method of the two spoons.

You can also give him food that he can eat with his hands. In this way, you will be actively stimulating his freedom regarding food. The food you give him must be firm so that the baby can grasp it with his hand but also soft and tender enough so that he can chew it before swallowing. The fact that he has teeth does not mean that he knows how to use them correctly and, in some cases, he can choke. By letting him experiment and giving him freedom with food, he will learn faster to feed himself.

Keep him under Supervision all the time when eating!

Allow your baby to take food with his hands or the spoon. Select chunks he can hold easily.

NEW CHALLENGES

It often happens that the baby finds it difficult to receive or try new tastes or textures. You have to give him time to get used to each new food. Without pressures or troubles soon, these small difficulties will be overcome. Let's see the most common ones.

1. **It expels more food than it swallows**. One possibility is that you have weaned the baby earlier than expected, but it may also be that he does not like the type of food you are giving him. You can start modifying (in tastes or textures) the food that you are usually incorporating into his diet. If this does not work, your baby may still not be prepared enough to start incorporating solids; in this case, it is convenient to wait and try again a few weeks later.

2. **When it seems that he does not like it.** It is possible that in the absence of eating habits for the child, it is difficult to start incorporating food. This situation can get them upset, irritable or even cause them to retch. One option is to dilute the food or puree in breast milk or formula of the second semester or water so that it is not so thick. You can also try offering small spoons of food.

3. **When your baby has no appetite, you should not force him to eat.** As with adults, the appetite in children is variable and changes constantly. If the baby does not have problems incorporating solids and suddenly stops eating or refuses food, it means that he is already satisfied. In the case of having doubts or being worried, consult with your pediatrician, who will surely weigh the child and identify if there is any possible inconvenience.

4. **When he is nauseous**. Your baby may feel nauseous if you are giving him

too much food or if you put lots of it in his mouth. Offer him food more slowly and in smaller portions. The important thing is not to get nervous or anxious since you will transmit this feeling to the baby and he will not want to eat. Do not force him to eat if he refuses; he may already be satisfied; if you force him to overeat, he can vomit easily.

5. If he does not want to incorporate liquids, It is important to keep in mind that the baby receives liquids in different ways and therefore does not face the risk of dehydration. If he refuses to drink water, it is because he is receiving enough from milk and purees.

Learning to feed by himself means a great progress in the small and intellectual development of your baby. It is fundamental that parents stimulate all of their attempts.

HOW TO SERVE FOODS:

Give him vegetables and fruits on small dices so the baby can take with his hands.

Cut the meat in small chunks, offer him slices of bread.

Change the way of cooking, sometimes grill it and sometimes use the oven.

Offer combined meals once they are tolerated individually.

Give him some meat daily (beef, chicken or fish). Ask your pediatrician if you consider a vegetarian diet for your baby.

Introduce your baby to the usage of the spoon.

Try to maintain a pleasant and peaceful environment.

THE PEDIATRIC DENTIST ADVICE

Parents and caregiver's oral health status has implications for the child's oral health. Remember that dental caries is an infection produced by microbes that are transmitted by adults when sharing cutlery, blowing food, cleaning the pacifier with their mouth, testing the temperature of the bottle or kissing them in the mouth.

The first consultation with the pediatric dentist must be done after 12 months. The hygiene is necessary, and you can do it with a brush or fingers without toothpaste.

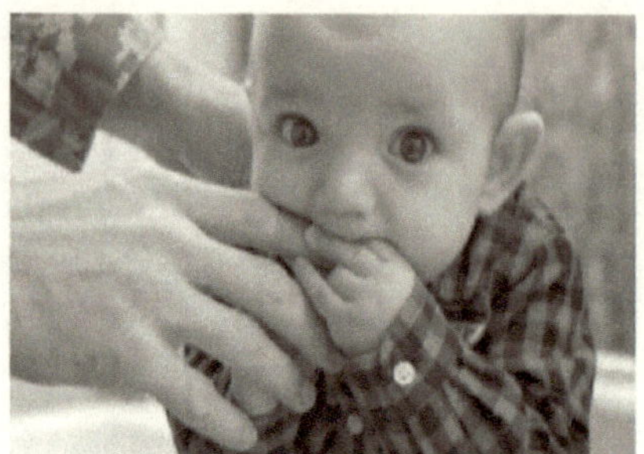

MOZZARELLA CHEESE BABY STICKS

🍼 9-12 months

🔺 6 servings

Ingredients

8 oz (200g) pasteurized Mozzarella (from cow's milk), cut into 8 finger-like strips.

2 eggs.

3 cups /10 Oz. (300g) Plain bread crumbs.

2 tomatoes

3 basil leaves

Directions

1. In a small bowl, whisk the egg.

2. Cut the cheese into finger-like strips, dip them with the eggs and then

roll in bread crumbs.

3. Repeat the operation with the eggs and bread crumbs 2 times for a better result.

4. Put the mozzarella sticks on the refrigerator (or 30 mins in the freezer) until hard.

5. For the sauce, process the peeled tomatoes (with no seeds), heat on a saucepan until you reduce the volume to ¼ of its original size. Add the basil leaves.

6. Place cheese sticks in a single layer on prepared baking sheet. Spray thoroughly with cooking spray. Bake 5-8 minutes, then turn and cook another 5-8 minutes on another side until golden and crispy. Allow cooling slightly before serving with the tomato sauce.

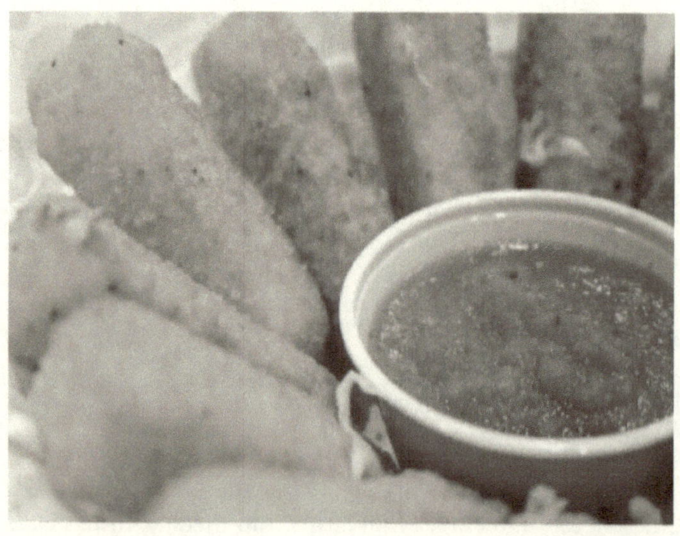

It's easier if you freeze the mozzarella sticks before dipping them into the eggs.

BANANA BREAD

🍼 9-12 months

🍽 4 servings

Ingredients

2 cups white whole-wheat flour

1 tablespoon plus 1⁄2 teaspoon baking powder, divided

1 teaspoon baking soda

3⁄4 teaspoon salt

1⁄2 cup applesauce

1⁄2 cup butter softened

2 tablespoons apple juice concentrate

1⁄3 cup agave nectar

1 teaspoon vanilla extract

4 ripe medium bananas.

Directions

1. Preheat oven to 350°F. Lightly oil a standard loaf pan.

2. In a medium bowl combine flour, 1 tablespoon baking powder, baking soda, and salt.

3. In a large bowl, combine applesauce with 1⁄2 teaspoon baking powder.

4. Add butter, apple juice concentrate, agave nectar, and vanilla to applesauce and mix well.

5. In a medium bowl, mash the bananas, mix bananas into wet ingredients.

6. Slowly mix dry ingredients into wet.

7. Pour batter into prepared loaf pan.

8. Bake 1 hour or until a toothpick inserted into the center of the loaf comes out clean.

9. Cool 10 minutes in the pan, then cool completely on cooling rack.

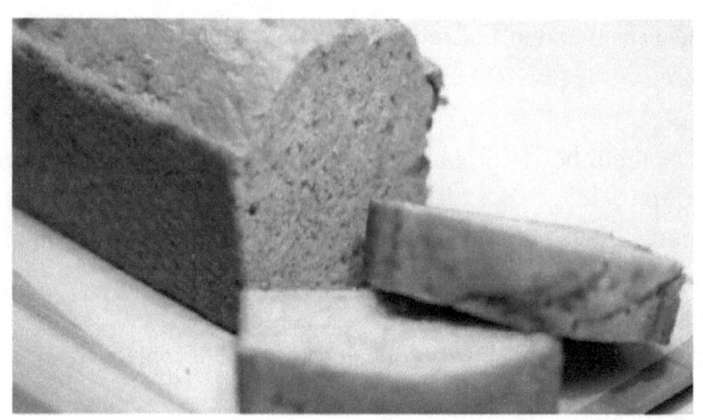

COD, CARROTS AND LEEK PUREE

🐘 9-12 months

🔔 2 servings

Ingredients

1 6-ounce (170g) Cod fillet. (or other white fish)

2 carrots peeled and chopped

1 leek, white and green parts only, chopped

½ cup boiled water (reserved), breast milk or formula.

Directions

1. In a medium saucepan, bring 2 inches of water to a boil over medium heat. Place the cod fillet, carrots, and leek into a steamer basket and steam for 15 minutes, covered. Let cool slightly.

2. Transfer all ingredients into a blender or food processor and blend until smooth, adding 1/4 cup of liquid at a time, until you have reached your desired consistency

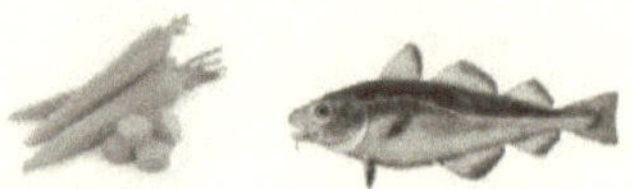

BABY BEEF STEW

🍼 9-12 months

🍽 2-4 servings

Ingredients

½ pound beef chuck boneless roast, cut into ½ inch cubes

2 Tsp olive oil

¼ small onion, chopped

1 Carrot or 10 Baby Carrots, peeled and chopped into 2-inch pieces

1 Medium Potato peeled and cut into 1-inch cubes

1 Cup water.

Directions

1. Heat the oil in a heavy bottom pot over medium/high heat.

2. Add the beef chunks and sear for 2-3 minutes on each side until brown.

3. Add the onions, carrots, potatoes, and water.

4. Stir the ingredients and bring to a boil.

5. Reduce the heat to low, cover and cook for 1 hour 15 minutes or until the beef and vegetables are tender.

6. Puree in a food processor until smooth or desired texture for your baby

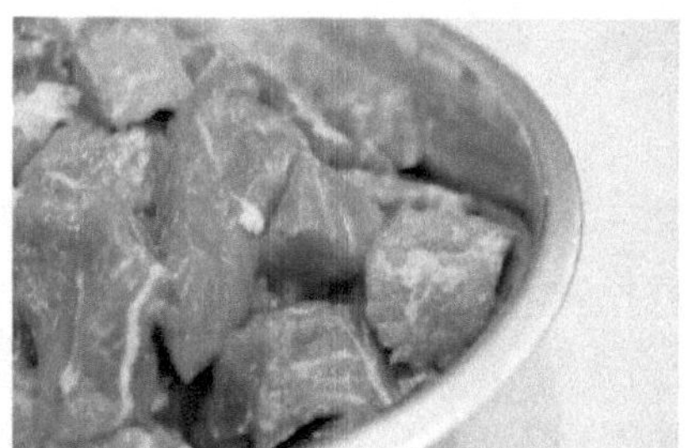

CREAMY BABY POTATO SOUP

9-12 months

6-8 servings

Ingredients

4 leeks, white and green parts only, chopped

2 tbsp of oil (30cc)

2 cups (500cc) of vegetable broth (homemade)

20 oz (600 g) of potatoes.

4 tbsp (80cc) of heavy cream.

Directions

1. Chop the leeks and the potatoes (clean them first)

2. Cook the leek for 2 minutes, add the broth and wait until it boils.

3. Add the potatoes and cook until they are soft.

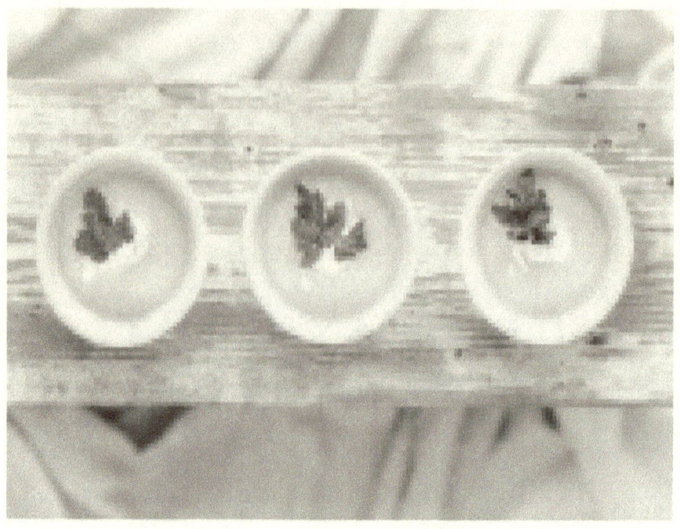

4. Process all, add the oil, the cream, mix and heat the soup.

CHICKEN BURGERS!

🐢 9-12 months

🍲 8-10 servings

Ingredients

3 organic chicken breasts (boneless and skinless)

2 leeks, white and green parts only

1 carrot chopped very small

1 egg yolk

1 cup of oatmeal (100g)

½ cup of plain bread crumbs (50g)

Olive Oil or vegetable cooking spray

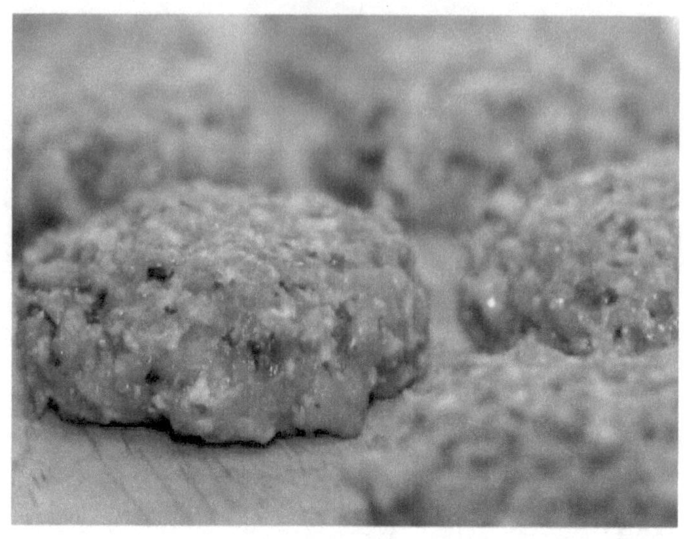

Directions

1. Mix all the ingredients and process them until you get a paste.

2. Prepare small burgers with the mix (or you can make some shapes).

3. Place them in a single layer on the prepared baking sheet. Spray thoroughly with cooking spray. Bake 20 minutes covered with an aluminum foil.

CHEESE SOUFFLÉ

🍼 9-12 months

🍽 4 servings

Ingredients

1/3 cup (40g) flour

3 tbsp. butter (40g)

1 cup (240 ml) milk.

3 large eggs (2 yolks, 3 whites)

2 tbsp. grated parmesan cheese

Directions

1. Preheat oven to 375º F (190ºC). Place a baking sheet on the middle rack in the oven. Butter 4 ramekins of 8-9 oz (230-250ml) capacity.

2. In a medium saucepan, melt the butter over medium-low heat. Add the flour and stir until smooth, and cook for about 1-2 minutes, until bubbling. Gradually stir in milk, until mixture is smooth. Bring to a boil, stirring constantly; cook and stir 2-3 minutes more or until thickened (bechamel sauce).

3. Remove from heat and stir in cheeses. Add 2 egg yolks, one at a time. Transfer mixture to a larger bowl and let cool slightly.

4. In a separate bowl whip 3 egg whites with a pinch of salt until stiff peaks form. Gradually fold the whipped whites into the cheese mixture.

5. Divide mixture evenly into the prepared ramekins. Sprinkle grated parmesan on top of each.

6. Place the ramekins onto the preheated baking sheet and bake for 25-30 mins until golden and puffed

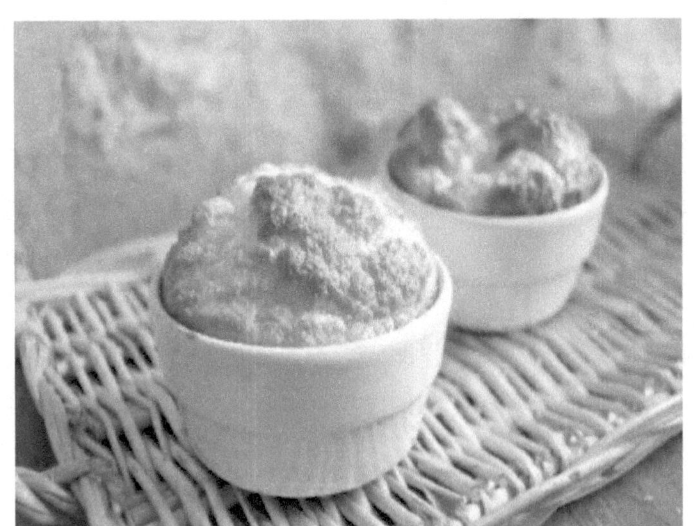

BROCCOLI &
CAULIFLOWER
CHEESE

9-12 months

4 servings

Ingredients

1 cup (4 oz/125 g) cauliflower florets, chopped into pieces small enough for your child to eat safely

1 cup (4 oz/125 g) broccoli florets, chopped into pieces small enough for your child to eat safely

1 tablespoon unsalted butter

1 tablespoon all-purpose flour

½ cup (4 fl. oz/125 ml) whole milk, plus more if needed

½ cup (2 oz/60 g) shredded mild white cheddar cheese.

1. Preheat oven to 375°F (190°C). Spray a small baking dish (just large enough to hold all the vegetables) with cooking spray or coat with butter.

2. Bring a saucepan half full of water to a boil over high heat. Add the broccoli and cauliflower and cook until tender, about 3 to 5 minutes. Drain and rinse under cold water; drain again. Pour the vegetables into the prepared baking dish.

3. Return the saucepan to medium heat and melt the butter. Whisk in the flour, let bubble for a minute or two, then slowly whisk in the milk. Let simmer for another minute, then sprinkle in the cheese, stirring until melted. If the sauce is too thick, add a tiny bit more milk. Pour the cheese sauce over the vegetables. Stir to combine.

4. Bake until browned and bubbling about 15 minutes. Let cool before serving. Cover and refrigerate for up to three days.

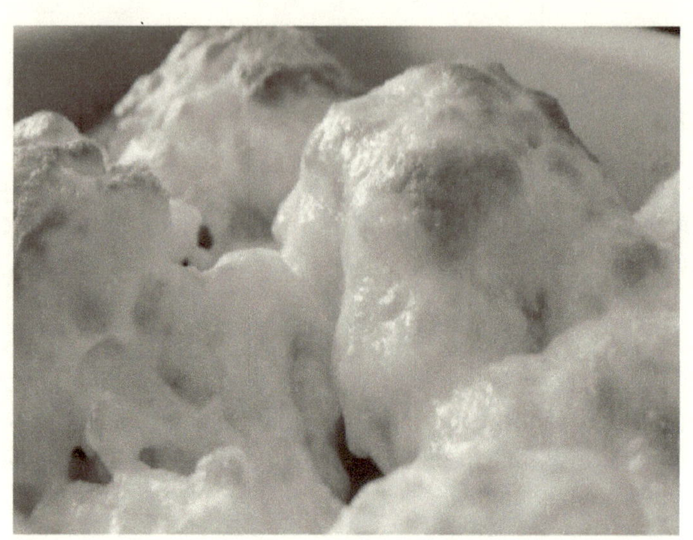

APPLE AND SWEET POTATO RÖSTI

9-12 months

2-3 servings

Ingredients

1 Big sweet potato.

1 green apple

2 tbsp. Butter (25g).

1 tbsp. oil

Directions

1. Preheat the oven to 220°C.

2. Grate the sweet potatoes and the green apple using the coarse side of the grater or a food processor.

3. Mix them with the liquid butter.

4. Divide the mixture into 4 and shape into rough cakes with your hands or place them into 3- or 4-inches Stainless Steel Cooking Rings (half-fill with the preparation).

5. Place on a large non-stick baking tray, and drizzle with the oil. Roast in the preheated oven for 25-30 minutes, or until golden brown and cooked through.

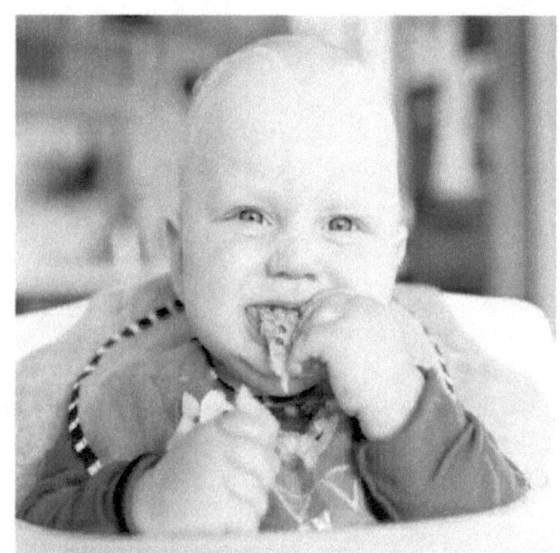

SPECIAL FRUIT SALAD

🐢 9-12 months

🍽 1 serving

Ingredients

1 oz (30g) Pear.

1 oz (30g) Orange.

1 oz (30g) Mandarine (or Mandarin Orange).

1 oz (30g) Banana (½ banana)

Directions

1. Peel an remove the seeds from the pear.

2. Remove the seeds and the white part of oranges.

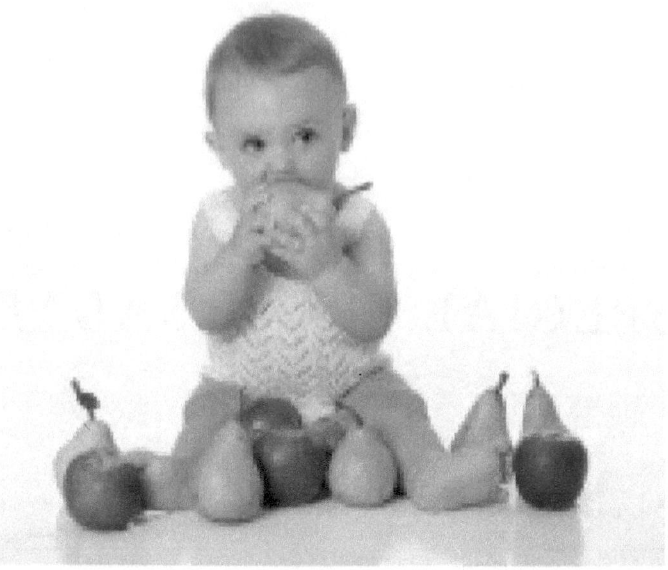

3. Peel and slice the banana

4. Prepare the dish by decorating it with the sliced fruits, so it becomes attractive to your baby.

ROASTED PEARS

9-12 months

4 serving

Ingredients

4 ripe pears (about 2 lbs.)

2 teaspoons olive oil.

Directions

1. Peel an remove the seeds from the pear.

2. Preheat the oven to 375°F.

3. Peel and core the pears; slice each into 8 wedges. Toss the pears with the olive oil. Spread them out on the baking sheet and roast for 30 minutes or until tender and lightly golden brown. Cool slightly.

You can Sprinkle the pears with some cinnamon if you desire.

Pears are generally softer so keep a watch as they may bake up faster

than you realize.

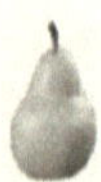

BABY'S FIRST BOLOGNESE

🍼 9-12 months

🔔 4-6 serving

Ingredients

7 oz (200g) lean mince meat

1 onion (chopped finely)

2 cups of fresh chopped tomatoes (400g)

½ celery stalk (chopped)

1 tbsp tomato puree

1 clove garlic (crushed)

1 tbsp olive oil

½ cup (50g) pasta (penne, shells, macaroni).

Directions

1. Heat the oil in a saucepan and add the chopped onions and crushed

garlic. Fry until onion is soft.

2. Add the mince and stir until the meat has browned.

3. Add the chopped tomatoes, tomato puree, and celery.
4. Stir until mixed thoroughly, then reduce heat slightly, cover and simmer for 20 minutes, stirring occasionally.

5. Cook pasta according to packet instructions, drain and serve mixed through the Bolognese sauce. You can decorate with basil leaves.

6. Mash or puree to desired consistency.

QUICK CHICKEN NUGGETS

9-12 months

4 serving

Ingredients

½ pound organic chicken breast

1 large egg

1 dash salt

½ cup plain bread crumbs.

2 tablespoon butter (unsalted).

1. Boil the chicken breast for 20 minutes in water

2. In a blender, blend cooked chicken breast, one egg, and salt.

3. Pack small balls of the meat mixture into cookie cutters and roll in bread crumbs.

4. Place them onto a cookie sheet. Drizzle with a little butter to make them crispier.

5. Bake at 400 degrees for about 10 minutes. Flip halfway through if you want both sides crispy.

PEA PANCAKES

🍼 9-12 months

🍽 4-8 serving (16 pancakes)

Ingredients

3 cups (400g) Frozen organic Peas

3 Eggs

1 ½ (180g) Self-raising flour

1 spring onion - chopped

1/3 cup (55g) Crumbled Feta Cheese

2 tbsp Chopped Parsley.

Directions

1. Boil the peas for 4 minutes and drain.

2. Add the flour, eggs, spring onion and half of the peas to a food processor and pulse until combined.

3. Fold through the remaining peas, feta cheese, and parsley

4. Fry tablespoons of the mixture in a little oil for approx. 2 minutes on each side until golden.

You can substitute self-rising flour with all-purpose flour and 1 tsp of baking powder.

If your kids don't like texture, then you can blend all the peas into the mixture.

SWEET POTATO FRIES

🐾 9-12 months

🍽 2-4 serving

Ingredients

Olive oil, for tossing

2 sweet potatoes, peeled, sliced into 1/3cm-thick slices, then 1/3cm-long strips, using a crinkle cut knife

Oil.

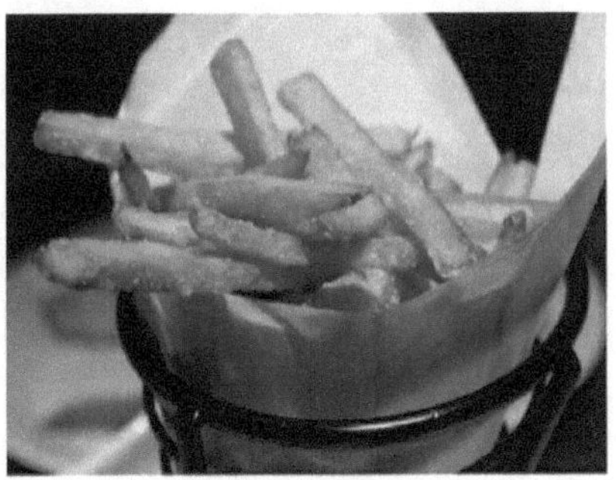

1. Preheat the oven to 400°F.

2. Line a sheet tray with parchment. In a large bowl, toss the sweet potatoes with just enough oil to coat.

3. Spread the sweet potatoes in a single layer on the prepared baking sheet, being sure not to overcrowd. Bake until the sweet potatoes are tender and golden brown, occasionally turning, about 20 minutes.

PARMESAN FISH FINGERS

🍼 9-12 months

🍽 4-6 serving

Ingredients

1 (500g) center-cut white fish fillet, about 9 inches (23cm) by 4 inches (10cm), skinned

½ cup (65g) plain flour

1/2 tsp fine sea salt

1/4 tsp freshly ground black pepper

3 egg whites

1 cup (90g) grated parmesan

1 cup (150g) plain bread crumbs

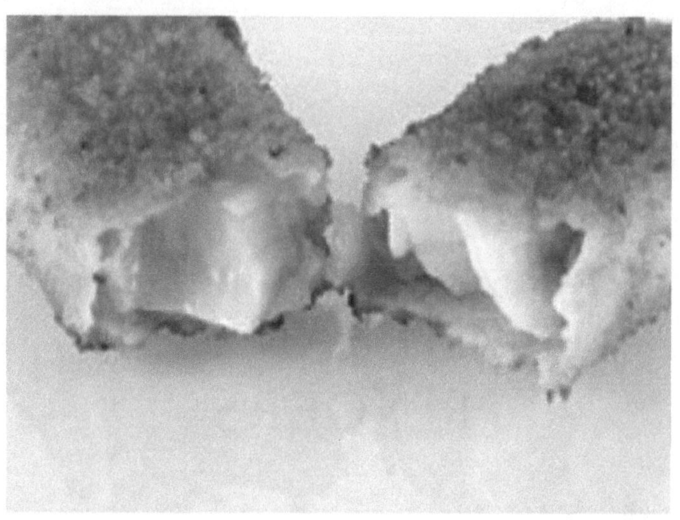

Directions

1. Preheat the oven to 450°F.

2. Rinse the fish fillet and pat dry with paper towels. Cut the fish in half to make two fillets each about 4 inches (10cm) by 5 inches (11.5cm). Starting on the longest edge, slice the fillets into 1-inch pieces. Lay the widest pieces, from the center and cut side down, and slice in half lengthways, so all the fingers are equally about 1inch by 1inch by 5 inches (11.5cm) in size.

3. Place the flour in a medium bowl and season with the salt and pepper. Place the egg whites in another bowl and beat until frothy, about 30 seconds. Combine the Parmesan and bread crumbs in a third bowl.

4. Coat the salmon fingers in the seasoned flour and pat to remove any excess. Dip the floured salmon in the egg whites and then into the Parmesan mixture, gently pressing the mixture into the fish.

5. Place the breaded salmon fingers on a slightly oiled baking tray. Drizzle with the olive oil. Bake for 15 to 20 minutes until golden brown.

You can dip them with the avocado dip in the next recipe.

AVOCADO DIP

🐢 9-12 months

🔔 Four serving

Ingredients

2 Avocados

¼ cup (30ml) Lemon juice (juice of 1/2 large lemon)

¼ cup (30ml) Olive Oil

1 tbsp finely Chopped parsley.

Directions

1. Add all ingredients to a food processor/blender and mix until smooth and creamy.

You can mash cottage cheese and avocado for a healthy "meal" or snack

Cheeses are typically offered to the non-allergic baby between eight and ten months of age. If your baby has a known or suspected dairy issue (either a milk protein or lactose intolerance) then you should wait to introduce cheese and another dairy when your infant is older

As always, you should consult baby's pediatrician about introducing cheese to your baby as generalities may not apply.

QUICK COUSCOUS WITH VEGGIES

9-12 months

1-2 serving

Ingredients

5 tbsp. (50g) Couscous

1 tsp rapeseed oil

½ tsp fresh lemon juice

1/8 cup (20g) frozen peas

¼ avocado (seed removed and diced)

½ tsp dried dill (optional)

½ carrot (small, chopped finely or grated)

Water.

Directions

1. Boil 2 cups of water.

2. In a bowl, combine the couscous, oil and lemon juice.

3. Pour ¼ cup (50ml) of boiling water over the couscous mixture and leave to soak for about 5 minutes.
4. Separate the grains with a fork.

5. Meanwhile, in a saucepan, add the carrots to boiling water, cook for about 4-5mins and then add the peas.

6. Cook for 3-4 minutes more until the vegetables are tender.

7. Drain and allow to cool.

8. Stir the avocado through the couscous and then mix with the veggies.

CHAPTER 5: BABY EATS THE FAMILY FOOD.

(1 -2 YEARS).

Once the year is over, your baby will have tripled his birth weight and begin to grow at a slower pace. He is already able to chew, eat things he takes with his hands and also drink with the cup. He can sit in his car seat and eat the same food as the rest of the family.

It is a good moment to establish the space of food as the place of dialogue, exchange and family encounter.

He will also learn to ask for a certain food. In the beginning, pointing it with his finger and then calling him by his name. And he will be aware that, if he does not like something, he can discard it or refuse to eat it. In this way, he will be starting to make decisions for himself.

THE HEALTHIEST FOOD

A healthy baby begins to spend more energy from the age of one. You will need to design a varied diet that provides him with the right amount of nutrients to guarantee his growth and the possibility to carry out activities. At this age, some babies may seem a bit overweight, but once they start walking and moving on their own, they lose weight rapidly. Don't forget that your baby will need a large supply of calories to help him develop the growth of his muscles, tissues, and bones.

In this way, fats will constitute the first concentrated source of fat-soluble vitamins A, D, E and K and essential fatty acids that the body does not produce. They will also allow the baby the correct development of the brain and nervous system. It is very important not to give low-fat or low-fat foods at this age.

Your baby will also need to consume around 500 cm^3 of milk daily, but in this case, you can already give him whole cow's milk fortified with iron. Try giving it to him in a cup so he can start giving up the bottle. At this time, he should not receive the nighttime milk drink. It is important not to incorporate a high fiber content in his diet because they are bulky and fill the stomach, and they do not provide the number of calories needed for this stage.

If your baby does not want to take the recommended 500 cm3 of milk per day, you can replace them during meals by giving him yogurt, white cheese, milkshakes, sauces or purees with milk among many other alternatives.

Fruits and vegetables are essential in your baby's balanced diet. It is ideal that you offer the child these foods both at breakfast (they can be pieces of banana or apple) and in the snack or lunch (in the form of sticks of celery, pieces of tomato). You can also incorporate them in snacks between meals, replacing cookies. Try to have some bread, cereals or potatoes at every meal; also, some fruit or vegetables and some milk, meat, fish or vegetables. These combined foods will give your baby everything he needs.

A GOOD TIME IN THE FAMILY

During this stage, your baby will already be able to eat with the rest of the family and the same food as them. In this period, where the baby's preferences are not fully developed or defined, it is easier to introduce new foods. You can give dishes that are striking for its texture, color, shape or decoration.

It is very important that you do not get angry with him if he refuses to eat the new foods and, above all, do not ever deny him the dessert or threaten to take it away from him. Try, however, prepare a nutritious dessert that compensates.

Family meals are also important as they allow you to coordinate the schedules and your baby will learn to behave at the table. If it is not possible to eat as a family, it is important that a brother or relative can accompany you. Your baby should have his cutlery and sit correctly at the table to feel like a member more

Also, it is recommended that you can, from time to time, share meals with friends or boys of your baby's age. In this way, you will find it more entertaining, and in some cases, you will be interested in eating foods that you do not usually eat just because you see another child doing it.

Recall that children acquire to a large extent the habits of the elderly.

If parents are not able to meet healthy habits, they cannot expect their children to acquire them. Try to reinforce hygienic habits before sitting down at the table – washing hands and face - as well as brushing teeth at the end of each meal.

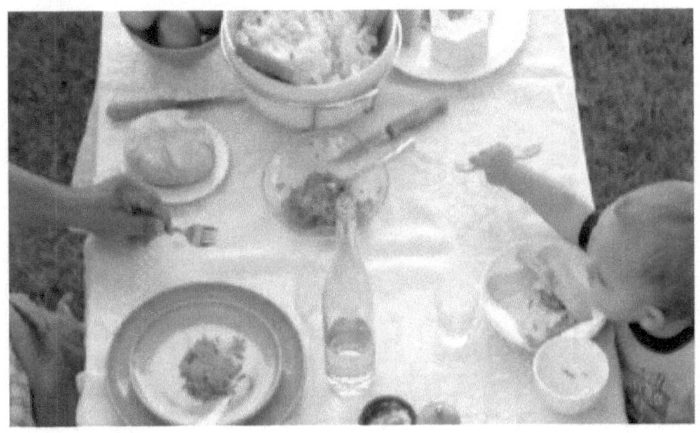

TO TAKE INTO ACCOUNT

Independence, ability and, why not, also the whims of the baby at mealtime can be disconcerting for some parents who are used to seeing their baby eat everything, very well and without saying anything. They should be alerted that this attitude change is normal at this stage of life. For this reason, you should not give more importance than they deserve to selectivity, lack of appetite or whims. This is where food becomes an element of negotiation between the mother and the child. The most appropriate behavior is a very calm reaction, not promoting or allowing tantrums at mealtime and not giving anything to your baby between meals.

If your baby does not want to eat more or leave part of the portion, it is better to allow it. At the next meal, he will eat more and with less tension.

THE PEDIATRIC DENTIST ADVISES

From 12 to 24 months the development and maturation of the masticatory system continue, and it will be completed in three months with the presence of twenty teeth in the mouth.

Avoid foods that contain a high percentage of carbohydrates, which adhere to the teeth and are slow dissolving. Oral hygiene in this period is done without toothpaste, by moistening the brush with water. The most important cleaning is the one done before going to sleep.

Dental erosion is a lesion produced by the acids in the diet that cause the irreversible loss of dental tissues. At present, this injury has increased due to changes in diets and the greater consumption of acidic juices and drinks. The citric, phosphoric, maleic and other acids contained in very frequently consumed beverages are responsible for this injury, which can be particularly destructive in children who ingest them in bottles, for prolonged periods close to the time of sleep. According to scientific evidence, the frequency with which they are ingested can be critical in the erosion process. At bedtime, the bottle should only contain water.

HUMMUS

🍼 1-2 years

🍽 1-2 serving

Ingredients

14.5 oz (400g) chickpeas previously boiled till tender

1 clove of garlic peeled and crushed

1 tablespoon lemon juice

¼ cup milk (can use water instead)

¼ cup tahini (sesame paste available near the jams and spreads in most supermarkets).

Directions

1. Combine all ingredients

2. Mash or puree with a blender until smooth.

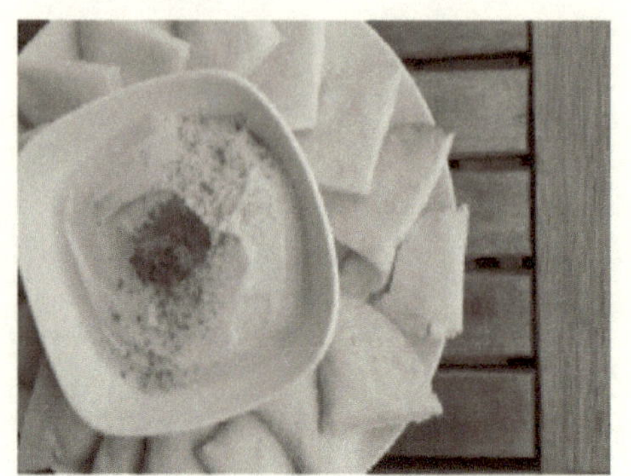

TODDLER COUSCOUS

🐢 1-2 Years

🍽 2-3 serving

Ingredients

1 cup unsalted water (or salt-reduced chicken stock)

¾ cup couscous

1 tablespoon olive oil

½ small onion, peeled and chopped

½ unpeeled organic zucchini, diced or grated whole

2 organic tomatoes chopped

1 cup (120g) cooked organic chicken, diced (or canned chickpeas.)

Directions

1. Place couscous in a separate bowl. Boil chicken stock or water. Pour chicken stock or water over couscous and let stand for about 6 minutes or until liquid is absorbed.

2. Heat oil in a saucepan over medium heat. Add onion and lightly fry for 2 minutes. Add zucchini and cook for about 4 minutes. Add tomato and cook for 1 minute.
3. Fluff the couscous with a fork and mix in the zucchini mixture and the chicken.

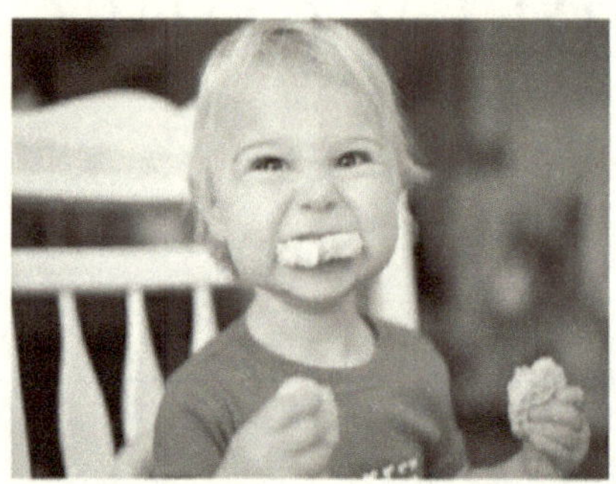

MUSHROOMS SANDWICH

🍼 1-2 years

🔔 2 serving

Ingredients

3 small mushrooms finely chopped

½ cup baked beans (or 130g can)

6 leaves spinach washed and chopped

4 slices wholemeal or multigrain bread

Olive oil or canola oil.

Directions

1. Microwave mushrooms on high for 30 seconds and drain excess moisture.

2. In a small bowl combine mushrooms, baked beans, and spinach.

3. Lightly spray sandwich maker with oil. Place two slices of bread on the base of the sandwich maker then divide the filling over the two slices. Top with two slices of bread and toast until heated through and golden brown.

You can replace mushrooms with other vegetables.

FISH BALLS

🐃 1-2 years

🛎 2-3 serving (12 balls)

Ingredients

2 potatoes peeled and chopped

½ onion, finely chopped

8.4 oz (180g) roasted tuna or salmon

½ medium carrot, peeled and grated

1 small zucchini grated

1 egg, lightly beaten

¼ cup of bread crumbs or flour

1 tablespoon vegetable oil.

Directions

1. Cook potato until tender. Drain and mash.

2. Mix potato, onion, tuna or salmon, carrot, zucchini, and egg together.

3. Shape the mixture into balls and roll in breadcrumbs or flour.

4. Heat oil in a non-stick frypan over medium heat. It can also be cooked in a 350°F oven.

5. Cook fish balls in batches until golden.

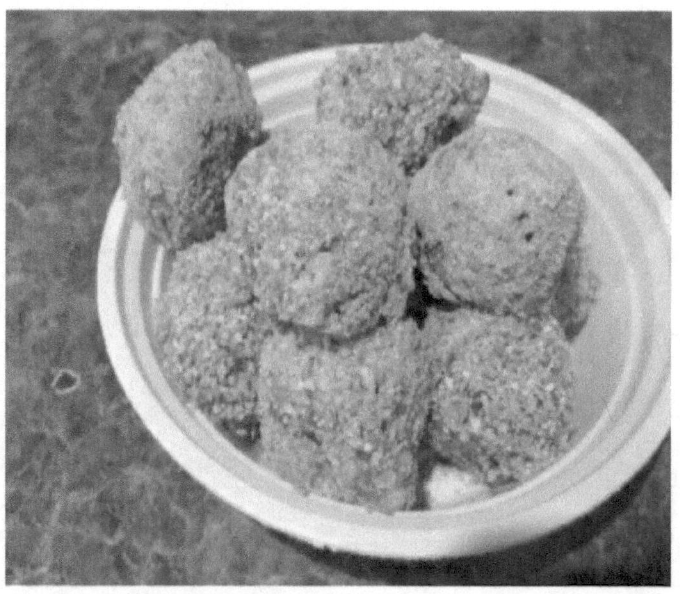

Fish is considered an important part of a heart-healthy diet. It's filled with nutrients the body needs for growth and maintenance. In general, pediatricians say parents can start introducing tuna at around six months of age.

Tuna offers protein without a high saturated fat content. It's also high in omega-3 fatty acids and B vitamins.

"Babies and young children require omega-3 fatty acids like DHA, available

in fish, for proper growth and development," says Ilana Muhlstein, R.D., a California-based dietitian. "Canned tuna is minimally processed and filled with good nutrition and simple ingredients."

The biggest concern with feeding babies with tuna is mercury exposure. Mercury is a metal that's found naturally and as a product of some manufacturing processes. When airborne mercury particles or vapor get into the water and come in contact with bacteria, it's turned into a substance that can be absorbed by fish living in that water.

People then eat the fish and absorb it themselves. Having too much mercury in your system can cause neurological problems.

The Federal Food and Drug Administration (FDA) advises avoiding:

- shark
- swordfish
- king mackerel
- tilefish

The above fish have the highest mercury content. But for children, the FDA says that two to three age-appropriate servings of a low-mercury fish source per week should be safe.

CHICKEN, VEGETABLE & PASTA SOUP

🚼 1-2 years

🍲 6 serving

Ingredients

10.5 oz (300g) skinless organic chicken breast, chopped

2 tablespoons olive oil

1 medium onion finely chopped

2 sticks chopped

2 carrots chopped

1 medium potato, chopped.

1 medium parsnip chopped

4 cups chicken stock, salt reduced

1 cup of water

½ cup macaroni pasta

1/3 cup grated cheese, to serve

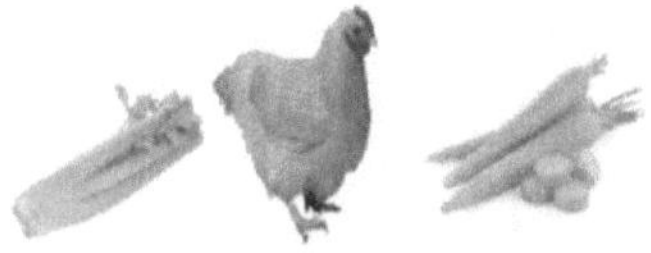

Directions

1. Heat 1 tablespoon of oil in large saucepan and cook chicken. Set aside.

2. Heat remaining oil in a saucepan over medium heat. Add onion and cook, stirring until soft.

3. Add celery, carrots, potato, and parsnip. Cook, occasionally stirring, for 5 minutes.

4. Pour in stock and water, cover and cook, occasionally stirring over medium heat for 25 minutes or until vegetables are tender.

5. Stir in pasta and cook, occasionally stirring, for 10 minutes or until pasta is tender.

6. Stir in chicken and heat through.

7. Serve warm sprinkled with grated cheese.

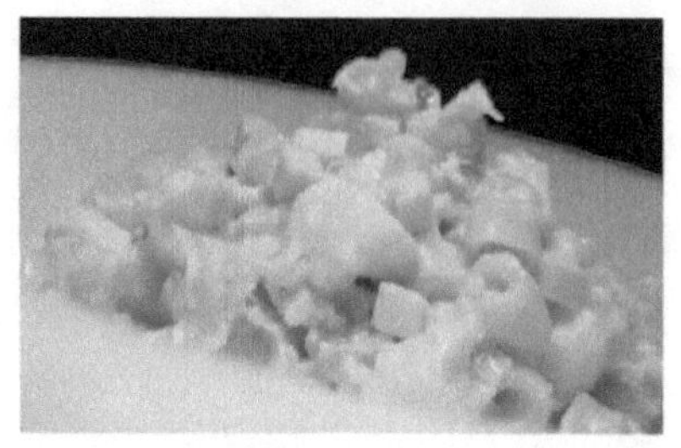

PIZZA DOUGH

🍼 1-2 years

🍽 4-6 serving

Ingredients

5oz (150g) wholemeal spelt flour

12oz (350g) strong white flour

1 ½ tsp dried fast action yeast

½ tsp salt

1 tbsp olive oil

Directions

1. To make the dough, put both flours into a large bowl, then stir in the yeast and salt. Make a well, pour in 400ml warm water and the olive oil and mix with a wooden spoon until you have a soft, fairly wet dough.

2. Bring together with a light knead in the bowl then turn onto a lightly floured surface and knead for 5 mins until smooth.

3. Cover with a tea towel and set aside. Leave the dough to rise if you have time, but it's not essential for a thin crust.

SPINACH PIZZA ROLLS

🍼 1-2 years

🍽 4-6 serving (12 rolls)

Ingredients

5 ounces (150g) spinach

1 tablespoon olive oil

13-16 ounces (350-450g) pizza dough (use previous recipe)

1 cup pizza sauce

2 cups shredded mozzarella cheese

1/4 cup grated Parmesan cheese

Directions

1. Preheat the oven to 400° F and grease a muffin tin. Warm the olive oil over medium heat in a skillet and cook the spinach just until wilted.

2. Remove from the heat and drain, pressing out all excess liquid. Use

your hands to stretch the dough into an 11×16-inch rectangle on a piece of parchment paper.

3. Spread enough pizza sauce over the dough to cover, then sprinkle on the spinach and mozzarella. Starting on one long side, roll the dough up carefully.
4. Use a serrated knife to cut into 12 even slices. Place each slice into a prepared muffin cup, sprinkle with Parmesan, and bake for 18-20 minutes until the dough is baked through, the cheese is melted, and the tops are golden.

5. Remove from pan, using a knife around the edges if needed, and let cool slightly before serving.

MINI PIZZAS

🐢 1-2 years

🔔 4-6 serving

Ingredients

16 oz (454g) of pizza dough (use previous recipe directions)

Tomato sauce of your choice

Mushrooms

Green pepper

Cherry tomatoes

1 8oz(226g) balls of Mozzarella

Fresh basil

Red onion

Red pepper

Kale or spinach

1 tbsp parmesan cheese (optional), for the crust

1. Preheat the oven to 485 degrees and put your pizza stone into the oven to heat up as the oven heats up (this is an important step as the stone can shatter if it's placed into the oven cold!)

2. On a floured surface, roll out your pizza dough so that it is about 1/2 an inch thin. You want it to be pretty thin because it will puff up in the oven!

3. Use a stainless-steel cup, glass cup or circular cookie cutter to create the same size circles of dough. You should be able to cut about 8 or 9 before you have to roll the dough up again to cut more.

4. To get the dough to stick together again, run it under water to get it wet enough so that it's sticky again, and roll it back out with some flour. Repeat with the cookie cutter, and you should end up with between 12-14 pieces of dough total.

5. Take the pizza stone out of the oven and place each little circle of dough onto the pizza stone. They will start to cook right away so place the whole stone into the oven right away and let the dough cook for 7-8 min.

6. Meanwhile, make sure all your toppings are ready, and cheese is grated.

7. Take the dough out of the oven (making sure it's slightly crisped on top and bottom). Top dough with tomato sauce, olive oil or whatever base you would like. Add cheese and toppings and put back in the oven for another 10-12 minutes, watching closely. Once the cheese is melted to your heart's desire, remove from the oven. You can sprinkle the crust with parmesan to get more crust. Before serving you can Sprinkle

chopped basil and allow the pizza to cool a few minutes.

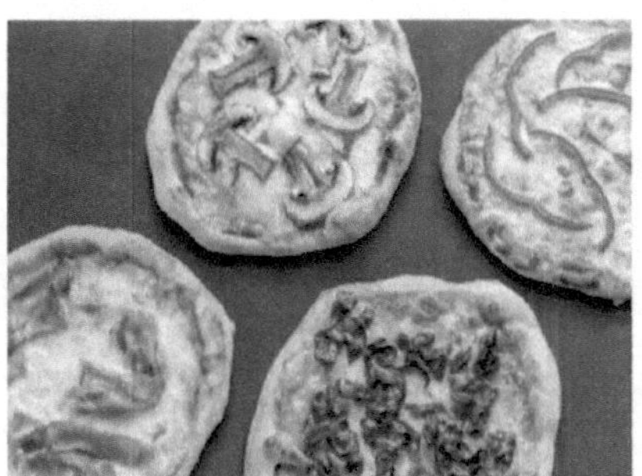

TODDLER MEATBALLS

🧒 1-2 years

🍽 4-6 serving

Ingredients

1/4 cup rolled oats

1/4 cup breadcrumbs

2-4 kale (or spinach) leaves, stems removed (or about 1/2 cup flat-leaf parsley leaves)

1 small onion peeled and roughly chopped

1 garlic clove peeled

1-pound (450g) ground organic beef

1/4 cup grated Parmesan cheese

1 egg

1. Preheat oven to 375 F. Line a rimmed baking sheet with foil and coat with nonstick spray.

2. Place the oats, breadcrumbs, kale, onion, and garlic in the bowl of a food processor — pulse to grind.

3. Add the rest of the ingredients and grind until thoroughly minced and uniform.

4. Form into 1-tablespoon-size meatballs and place on the prepared baking sheet.

5. Bake for about 18 minutes, or until brown and cooked. Drain on paper towels if necessary.

6. You can serve them alone, with some tomato (or his favorite) sauce, with your baby pasta.

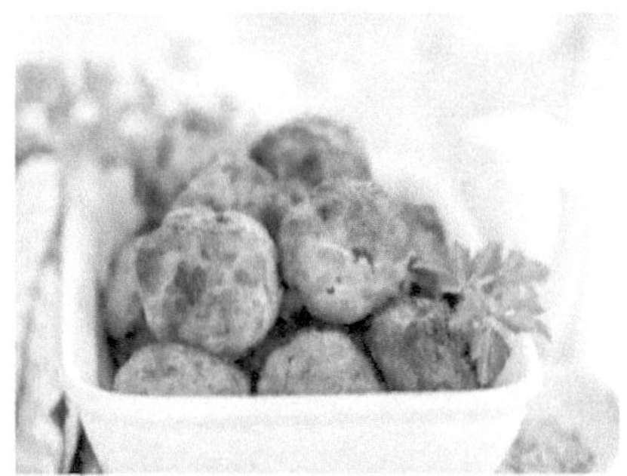

SWEETCORN & SPINACH FRITTERS

🐾 1-2 years

🍚 4 serving (12 fritters)

Ingredients

1 8.5oz (214g) can organic no-salt sweet corn, drained

1/2 cup baby spinach (or kale) leaf

1 small garlic clove crushed

1 spring onion chopped

½ cup (65g) plain flour

½ tsp baking powder

1 egg

1/5 cup (50ml) milk

1 tsp oil, for frying

Directions

1. Pulse all the ingredients except the oil in a food processor until fairly but not completely smooth.

2. Heat a little oil in a frying pan until hot and dollop four spoonfuls of the mixture into the pan leaving space around them. Fry for just under 1 min on each side until lightly golden.

3. When you flip the fritter, flatten with a spatula to ensure even cooking the whole way through.

4. Cook in three batches, placing the cooked fritters on a plate covered with kitchen roll.

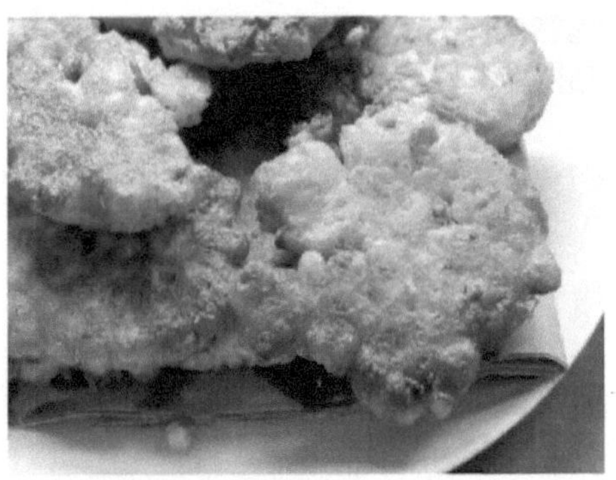

FISH & PASTA

1-2 years

2-4 serving

Ingredients

1 clove garlic minced

2 tablespoons olive oil

1-pound white fish (such as haddock, monkfish, or cod), cut into 2-inch chunks

½ cup vegetable broth

¼ cup of water

1 tablespoon chopped fresh basil (or flat parsley or cilantro)

¼ teaspoon dried oregano

½ pound whole wheat pasta

Lemon wedges (optional)

Grated parmesan cheese (optional)

1. In a 2-quart saucepan sauté the garlic in the oil for 1 minute.

2. Add fish, broth, water, basil, and oregano. Cover and simmer for 10 minutes.

3. While the fish simmers, cook the pasta according to package instructions.

4. Remove fish from heat and stir gently so as not to break up the fish too much.

5. Drain the pasta, put it in a large bowl, and pour all the fish with its cooking liquid over the pasta. Add a squeeze of lemon juice and toss with grated cheese.

CORN MUFFINS

🐛 1-2 years

🔺 2-4 serving

Ingredients

½ cup all-purpose flour

½ cup cornmeal

2 teaspoons baking powder

½ teaspoon salt

2 tablespoons sugar

½ cup milk

1 egg

2 tablespoons melted butter

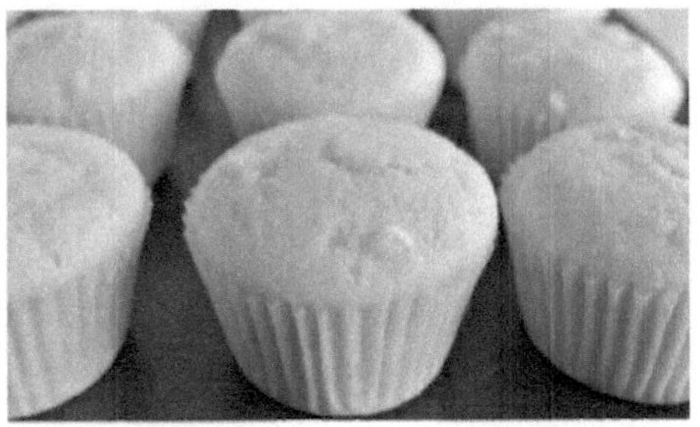

Directions

1. Preheat oven to 425°F.

2. Grease a muffin pan or use paper liners.

3. Combine flour, cornmeal, baking powder, salt, and sugar.

4. Form a well in the center of the flour mixture and add milk, egg, and butter. Stir by hand just until the wet and dry ingredients are blended.

5. Fill each muffin cup about two-thirds full. Bake 15–20 minutes, until the tops are golden brown.

SUGAR FREE COOKIES

🐾 1-2 years

🍲 6 serving

Ingredients

1/4 cup – coconut oil

2 medium – organic banana

1 large – egg

1 teaspoon – vanilla extract

1/4 teaspoon – cinnamon

1 3/4 cup – organic oats, dry

1/4 cup – raisins, seedless

Directions

1. Preheat oven to 350ºF. Lightly grease baking sheets and set aside. If coconut oil is in a solid state, heat gently until just melted.

2. Mash bananas; add to coconut oil and mix well. Fork-whisk in the egg and vanilla.

3. Stir in the oats, cinnamon, and raisins until combined.

4. Spoon the dough onto the baking sheets (you'll make 12-14 cookies.)

5. Bake for 15-18 minutes or until slightly golden. Serve warm, or room temperature. Refrigerate or freeze leftovers.

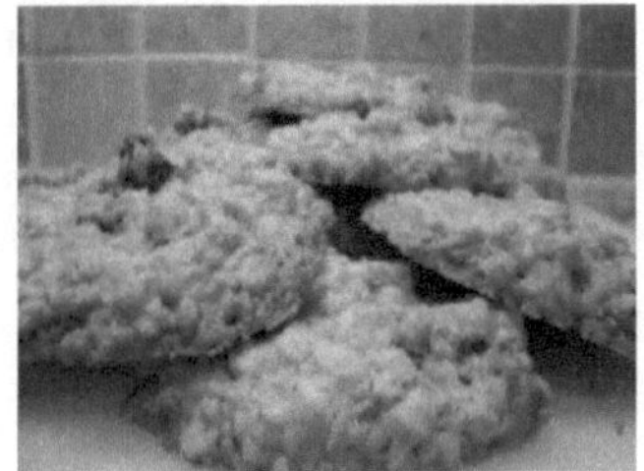

CHAPTER 6: HOW TO SHOP

From the year, your child's diet opens to a new world of flavors and textures, leading to doubts about which products are best suited for the child.

When making your shopping arrangements, organization is the key

There is no need to go shopping every day. Organize the menus weekly; this way you will not go wrong in quantities, and you will make sure that there is no lack of variety in the diet.

Make a weekly meal plan

Plan the menus throughout the week: this way the meals will be balanced, and you will avoid leftovers.

When shopping, keep in mind the days that food will be kept at home. Fruit and vegetables will be optimally maintained for about four days; then they will lose nutrients; the meat, about three days (except the minced, which should be consumed within 24 hours). And the fish cannot stand more than two days.

If you cannot go shopping very often, freezing is a good solution in which food will not lose nutrients. The exception is the fruit porridge: you should consume it at the moment and do not save what the leftovers.

ORGANIC FOOD

I recommend you buy organic food whenever you can because it will be better for your baby's health as well as the environment.

Surely, if you are a good observer, you will notice that fresh products tastes better than those that come from faraway places or have been subjected to chemical processes, not to mention the best-preserved nutrients due to the absence of pesticides or artificial preservatives.

Check with the local neighbors which is the nearest farm where you can buy this type of food. Even sometimes you can come to a fixed monthly agreement to be sure you always have the best things for the children. Local markets are a very good option.

Organic foods carry no antibiotics or growth hormones and are free of conventional pesticides, synthetic fertilizer, bioengineering, and irradiation.

It is good to know the data on organic and non-organic products, helping you make informed and healthy decisions.

Nutrition: Organic foods have different nutritional values. Some are more nutritious than their non-organic versions. Others have the same value. For example, organic fruits and vegetables may have more minerals, due to how they are grown. In contrast, organic snacks, such as cookies or ice cream, do not contain extra nutrition.

Artificial ingredients: This is the main difference between organic and non-organic foods. Growth hormones, synthetic ingredients, and pesticides are common in the food industry. They could cause long-term effects on health. It is believed that the consumption of organic foods can reduce the risk of future health problems.

Taste: Organic foods do not have preservatives. Local producers buy them, so they tend to be fresher. Also, they do not have chemicals and artificial flavors, so they have a more natural flavor. An organic label does not guarantee a better aspect or freshness, but you may discover that they taste better. Try organic products and organic dairy products to see if you prefer their flavor.

Environment: Organic agriculture is destined to be good for the environment. It helps reduce pollution, save water and resources and reduce soil erosion. Organic farmers do not use pesticides that can harm animals and plants. They also provide livestock with more humane living conditions. Organic foods are often sold in local stores, reducing the contamination of shipment throughout the country, and supporting local industries.

Duration: Organic products usually do not last as long as non-organic ones, because they do not have preservatives. Food, especially agricultural products, can spoil faster.

Cost: You may have noticed that organic foods are more expensive than non-organic foods. This is due to the higher cost of organic agriculture, as well as limited supplies. As more people use organic products, prices tend to decrease, as it is happening in the areas where people buy organic products more frequently.

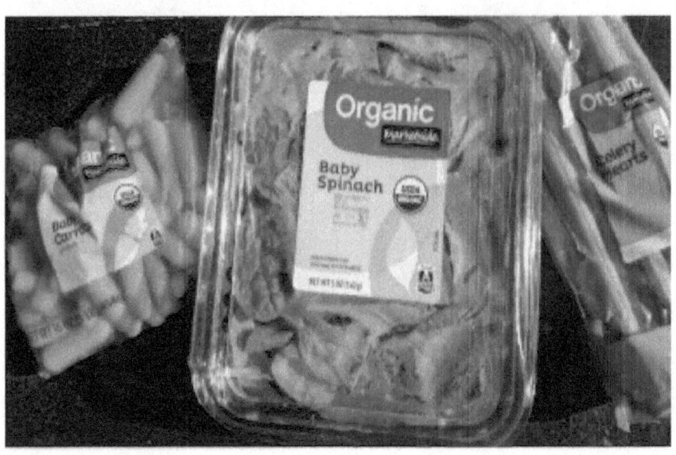

Organic Labeling

Food must meet certain standards to carry the organic label. Farmers, businesses and food products must be inspected and certified.

The USDA has several different "organic" labels. You may encounter the following:

100% organic means that the product you are buying has been produced and processed using approved methods and organic ingredients. You can frequently see this label in single-ingredient items, such as fruits or eggs.

Organic Products contain at least 90% organic ingredients.

Made of organic products, they contain at least 75% organic ingredients.

Other common labels are natural, sustainable, and grass-fed. The USDA does not define or control these terms officially. There is no guarantee that products with these labels follow the same rules.

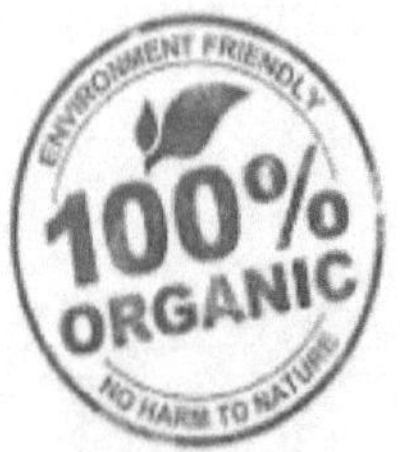

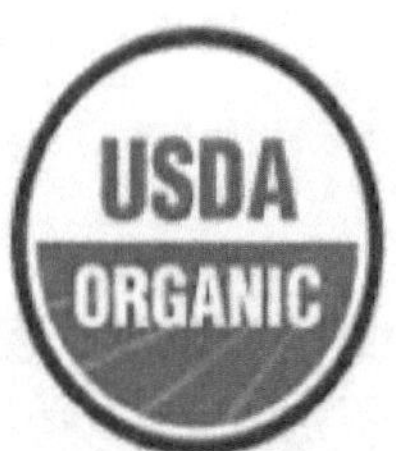

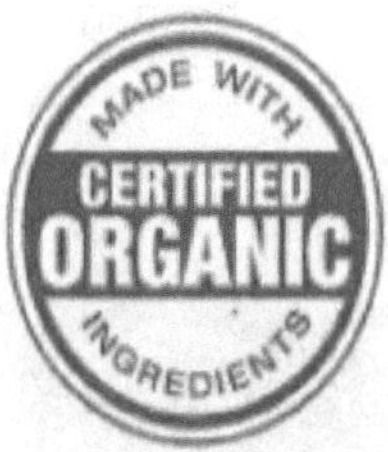

CHOOSE SEASONAL PRODUCTS

Fruits and vegetables should be seasonal to optimize nutrients, In summer, for instance, zucchini, carrot or pumpkin are at an excellent time.

Spring

Apples, Apricots, Asparagus, Avocados, Bananas, Broccoli, Cabbage, Carrots, Celery, Collard Greens, Garlic, Kale, Kiwifruit, Lemons, Lettuce, Limes, Mushrooms, Onions, Peas, Pineapples, Radishes, Rhubarb, Spinach, Strawberries, Swiss Chard, Turnips.

Summer

Apples, Apricots, Avocados, Bananas, Beets, Bell Peppers, Blackberries, Blueberries, Cantaloupe, Carrots, Celery, Cherries, Corn, Cucumbers, Eggplant, Garlic, Green Beans, Honeydew Melon, Lemons, Lima Beans, Limes, Mangos, Okra, Peaches, Plums, Raspberries, Strawberries, Summer Squash, Tomatillos, Tomatoes, Watermelon, Zucchini

Fall

Apples, Bananas, Beets, Bell Peppers, Broccoli, Brussels Sprouts, Cabbage, Carrots, Cauliflower, Celery, Collard Greens, Cranberries, Garlic, Ginger, Grapes, Green Beans, Kale, Kiwifruit, Lemons, Lettuce, Limes, Mangos, Mushrooms, Onions, Parsnips, Pears, Peas, Pineapples, Potatoes, Pumpkin, Radishes, Raspberries, Rutabagas, Spinach, Sweet Potatoes & Yams, Swiss Chard, Turnips, Winter Squash.

Winter

Apples, Avocados, Bananas, Beets, Brussels Sprouts, Cabbage, Carrots, Celery, Collard Greens, Grapefruit, Kale, Kiwifruit, Leeks, Lemons, Limes, Onions, Oranges, Parsnips, Pears, Pineapples, Potatoes, Pumpkin, Rutabagas, Sweet Potatoes & Yams, Swiss Chard, Turnips, Winter Squash

Source usda.gov

In today's globalized markets you can always get some of these products in the opposite season as they are imported from a different hemisphere. Consuming local, seasonal products you are offering your family a healthier option, helping protect the environment and supporting your local farmers and shops.

Be careful as this list is only to orientate you, and not all these products may be adequate for your baby age.

CHAPTER 7: MEASURING

METRIC CONVERSION GUIDE

Conversion guide

1 tablespoon (tbsp)	3 teaspoons (tsp)
1/16 cup =	1 tablespoon
1/8 cup =	2 tablespoons
1/6 cup =	2 tablespoons + 2 teaspoons
1/4 cup =	4 tablespoons
1/3 cup =	5 tablespoons + 1 teaspoons
3/8 cup =	6 tablespoons
1/2 cup =	8 tablespoons

2/3 cup =	10 tablespoons + 2 teaspoons
3/4 cup =	12 tablespoons
1 cup =	48 teaspoons
1 cup =	16 tablespoons
8 fluid ounces (fl. oz)	1 cup
1 pint (pt.) =	2 cups
1 quart (qt) =	2 pints
4 cups =	1 quart
1 gallon (gal) =	4 quarts
16 ounces (oz) =	1 pound (lb.)
1 milliliter (ml) =	1 cubic centimeter (cc)
1 inch (in) =	2.54 centimeters (cm)

Source: United States Dept. of Agriculture (USDA).

U.S. to Metric

CAPACITY		WEIGHT	
1/5 teaspoon	1 milliliter	1 oz	28 grams
1 teaspoon	5 ml	1 pound	454 grams
1 tablespoon	15 ml		
1 fluid oz	30 ml		
1/5 cup	47 ml		
1 cup	237 ml		
2 cups (1 pint)	473 ml		
4 cups (1 quart)	0.95 liter		
4 quarts (1	3.8 liters		

gal.)

Metric to U.S.

CAPACITY		WEIGHT	
1 milliliter	1/5 teaspoon	1 gram	0.035 ounce
5 ml	1 teaspoon	100 grams	3.5 ounces
15 ml	1 tablespoon	500 grams	1.10 pounds
100 ml	3.4 fluid oz	1 kilogram	2.205 pounds = 35 ounces
240 ml	1 cup		
1 liter	34 fluid oz = 4.2 cups = 2.1 pints = 1.06 quarts = 0.26		

	gallon		

OVEN TEMPERATURE

Fahrenheit	Celsius	Gas Mark	Terminology
275° F	140° C	1	Very Cool / Slow
300° F	150° C	2	Cool or Slow
325° F	165° C	3	Warm
350° F	177° C	4	Moderate
375° F	190° C	5	Moderate
400° F	200° C	6	Moderately Hot
425° F	220° C	7	Hot
450° F	230° C	8	Hot
475° F	245° C	9	Hot
500° F	260° C	10	Very Hot

These conversions are approximate for Fahrenheit, Celsius, and gas marks.

COOKING COMMON ABBREVIATIONS

Term	Description
t	teaspoon
tsp	teaspoon
T	tablespoon
Tbsp	tablespoon
c	cup
oz	ounce
pt	pint
qt	quart
Gal	gallon
Lb	pound
Dice	Cut into very small cubes.

Fillet	A cut of meat or fish without skin or bones.
Puree	Mixed in a tabletop blender or with a hand blender to a smooth consistency.
Mash	Mashed with a spoon or fork until only soft lumps remain
Stir fry	Stir with a small amount of oil over high heat for a short time
Boil	When bubbles reach the surface and break at a temperature of 212ºF (100ºC)
Simmering	When small bubbles form slowly and collapse below the surface at the temperature of 180ºF (80ºC–85ºC)

WEIGHTS OF COMMON INGREDIENTS IN GRAMS

Ingredient	1 cup	3/4 cup	2/3 cup	1/2 cup	1/3 cup	1/4 cup	2 Tbsp
Flour, all-purpose (wheat)	120 g	90 g	80 g	60 g	40 g	30 g	15 g
Flour well sifted all-purpose (wheat)	110 g	80 g	70 g	55 g	35 g	27 g	13 g
Sugar, granulated cane	200 g	150 g	130 g	100 g	65 g	50 g	25 g
Confectioner's sugar (cane)	100 g	75 g	70 g	50 g	35 g	25 g	13 g
Brown sugar packed firmly	180 g	135 g	120 g	90 g	60 g	45 g	23 g
Cornmeal	160 g	120 g	100 g	80 g	50 g	40 g	20 g

Corn starch	120 g	90 g	80 g	60 g	40 g	30 g	15 g
Rice, uncooked	190 g	140 g	125 g	95 g	65 g	48 g	24 g
Macaroni, uncooked	140 g	100 g	90 g	70 g	45 g	35 g	17 g
Couscous, uncooked	180 g	135 g	120 g	90 g	60 g	45 g	22 g
Oats, uncooked quick	90 g	65 g	60 g	45 g	30 g	22 g	11 g
Table salt	300 g	230 g	200 g	150 g	100 g	75 g	40 g
Butter	240 g	180 g	160 g	120 g	80 g	60 g	30 g
Vegetable shortening	190 g	140 g	125 g	95 g	65 g	48 g	24 g

Chopped fruits and vegetables	150 g	110 g	100 g	75 g	50 g	40 g	20 g
Nuts chopped	150 g	110 g	100 g	75 g	50 g	40 g	20 g
Nuts, ground	120 g	90 g	80 g	60 g	40 g	30 g	15 g
Bread crumbs, fresh, loosely packed	60 g	45 g	40 g	30 g	20 g	15 g	8 g
Bread crumbs, dry	150 g	110 g	100 g	75 g	50 g	40 g	20 g
Parmesan cheese grated	90 g	65 g	60 g	45 g	30 g	22 g	11 g

ABOUT THE AUTHOR

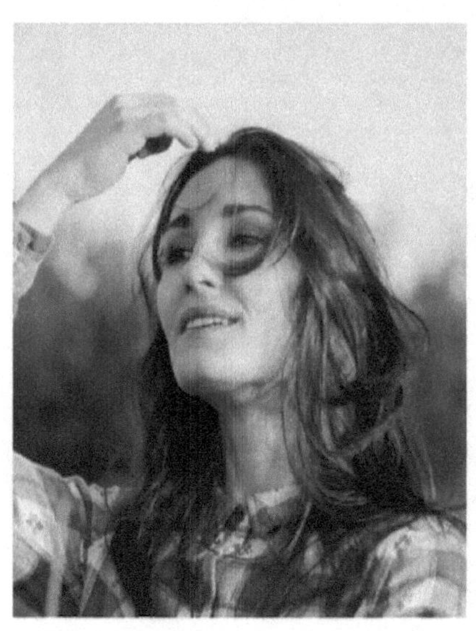

AUTHOR NAME is RUSTY COVE-SMITH

Find out more at amazon.com/author/rustycove

Or visit https://gimbooks.info/team/rusty-cove-smith/